UNCURSING THE DARK

Uncursing the Dark

Treasures from the Underworld

Betty De Shong Meador

Chiron Publications • *Asheville, North Carolina*

www.chironpublications.com

Library of Congress Catalog Card Number: 92-23029

Printed in the United States of America.
Editing and book design by Siobhan Drummond.
Cover design by Mercedes Santos.
Cover art by Julie Burleigh.

Library of Congress Cataloging-in-Publication Data:

Meador, Betty De Shong, 1931–

Uncursing the dark: treasures from the underworld / Betty De Shong Meador.
p. cm.
Includes English translations of The descent of Inanna to the underworld and other Sumerian texts.
Cover title.
Includes bibliographical references and index.
ISBN 978-1-63051-523-2
1. Initiation rites. 2. Initiation rites—Mythology. 3. Women—Psychology. 4. Goddess religion. 5. Feminist poetry. I. Descent of Inanna to the underworld. English. 1992. II. Title.
GN483.3.M43 1992
305.4—dc20 92-23029
CIP

ISBN 978-0-933029-65-1

For Ross, Liz, and Mary

Contents

Preface

On a summer night in the late 1930s my family was driving down a two-lane country road somewhere in East Texas. We must have been almost to our destination, for my father was relaxed, in a rare good mood, not rushing anywhere. He pulled over to the side of the road, and we all piled out to look at the rising full moon. A flat grassy field, still visible in the fading evening light, stretched in front of us. The moon rose far away over a line of black hills in the distance. It was creamy gold and huge just above the hills. We watched it shrink and turn white higher in the sky.

My father challenged us to find the man in the moon. Everyone, my parents, my older sister, even my little brother, pointed enthusiastically and beamed back to the moon a broad smile. I could not for the life of me see the man in the moon. My father patiently led my eager eyes across the shadows, naming each bulge one of the moon man's features. He would not come into view. Instead I saw a woman sitting, slightly leaning over something in her lap which I imagined to be knitting or sewing of some kind. "See!" I said, relieved I could see something. "There is a woman in the moon!" Try as they did to find my picture, no one in my family could see her.

This incident stamped itself vividly in my memory. Looking back I wonder through what lens my eyes focused so that I saw the woman, not the man, in the moon. Was the psyche of that eight- or ten-year-old child already in the grip of the archetype of the feminine so that some elemental pattern of perception brought forth the woman in the moon? Or is the archetypal feminine a natural element present in the instinctual makeup of any little girl? Whatever the answer may be, I saw with a given perception that was different from my family. I don't remember feeling left out or deficient in any way. In spite of what they said, I was certain there was a woman in the moon.

The essays in this book were written over a twenty-year period, and each one, in its own way, is an attempt to give expression to the archetype of the feminine. As a Jungian analyst, I subscribe to Jung's view of archetypal psychology. The archetypes, he says, are innate potential patterns, any one of which may constellate in a person's psyche and powerfully shape that person's way of being and perceiving the world. The archetypes are intimately connected to human instinct and are an inborn potential just as is instinct. While instinct drives and shapes how we behave at the most basic, primary level, archetype is the expression of instinct by which we apprehend meaning through the emotions that the instinctual drive mobilizes and through the images and fantasies that instinct triggers. The archetype, Jung says, "might suitably be described as the *instinct's perception of itself* or as the self-portrait of the instinct" (1919, par. 277). That is, the most primary emotions and images which convey how a person feels and thinks are archetypal signals from instinctual drives. A little girl in the grip of her own femaleness, her worldview configured by the biological/instinctual fact of being female, might very well see the woman, not the man, in the moon. Not every little girl is caught in the archetype of the feminine. However, this archetype is one which might easily constellate in the psyche of a young female child. The pattern of femaleness, informed by instinct and biology and individual circumstance and a hundred thousand years of evolution of the human female animal, might very well dominate the way she approaches the world.

To whatever extent the archetypal feminine shaped my early life, that worldview was challenged by a strong, domineering father and by the prevalence of masculine control in the culture of a small Texas town. The sequence of having one's innate sense of self challenged by conflicting beliefs of family or culture is not unusual. All of us are born into the molding demands of a particular society. The individuality we bring into the world at birth frequently bumps up against an inhospitable culture. This conflict becomes the drama of individuation as the innate self strives for full realization against the demands of cultural adaptation.

Outwardly thrown about by this conflict, I managed to respect the authenticity of the feminine as it manifested in dreams and life events. Somewhere in the middle of the twenty years these essays span, I came across the myth of Inanna's descent to the underworld. This myth tells an archetypal story of the primacy of the primordial, natural, instinctual feminine over the world of culture. The myth seemed to me the very substructure of the meaning of femaleness, the rock-bottom facts of women's relationship to the primal material world.

I discovered that this myth in one form or another had been at the heart of ritual practice for women for thousands of years, reaching back into Neolithic and possibly into Paleolithic time. A ritual of such duration must carry a fundamental and essential meaning crucial to women's understanding of themselves. The myth discloses an archetypal pattern of opposites. On the one hand, the woman descendant is the highly civilized culture bearer; on the other, at the bottom of the underworld, she is a single human animal, separate and alone with only her instinctual needs to guide her. For aeons, women placed this mythic pattern at the heart of their ritual observation. Yearly, in enactments of descent, they renewed their devotion to the primordial forces that infuse all matter with life and drastically determine our fate.

For many women familiar with this myth, the word *descent* immediately conjures up periods of crisis, depression, loss, tragedy, or madness. A descent, in popular psychology, is a down-going excursion away from the intact emotions of "normal" life, a ride on waves of disorientation, despair, and chaotic turmoil. The hope, and sometimes the goal, is to get out of the downward spiral as fast as possible.

I do not intend to minimize the suffering women endure in periods of descent. Instead, I wish to revise our understanding of descent's meaning. We have lost the ritual enactment which served to orient us during such periods. With our ritual meaning gone, we flounder, mapless and rudderless, at the mercy of tides of emotion.

Consider the two mythological versions of the descent to the underworld which appear in this book. One is Inanna's descent, a myth from 3500 B.C. or before; the second is the Thesmophoria, a Greek ritual from the first millennium B.C. In both versions, the goddess or the women who descend to the underworld return transformed. In each case, the one who descends from the upper world of cultural imperatives and forms discards these and stands naked before the ruler of the great below, a primordial being who endows all matter with a highly determined process of growth and decay. The descendant is shaken when she faces in her nakedness the absolute authority of she who turns the very wheel of life and death. Her hard won adaptation to culture means very little in the face of she who controls life itself. After such an experience the woman returns profoundly reoriented. Her devotion now is to primary being, the life process which breathes its inevitable course through all matter. The transformed woman reenters ordinary life within her own culture, but beneath her obligations to the culture, she remains aware of the ruling ebb and flow of nature's vital process. The dark stream of inevitable process maintains its constant course in the backwaters of her mind.

Until the past two thousand years, women have kept ritual watch on the deep, silent workings of nature. Ancient women assigned themselves the task of bearing consciousness of the profundity of life coursing through matter and kept that vigil through rituals based on the descent myth. Indeed, women's performance of a ritual watch on unpredictable nature may have generated the beginnings of culture itself. Our ancestors were burdened with the task of creating ritual forms through which they could experience and relate to the awesome, potentially overwhelming, potentially fragmenting powers of nature. Judy Grahn in her book, *Blood, Bread, and Roses* (in press), says that rituals pertaining to menstruation, woman's constant reminder of inevitable autonomous process, were the first conscious enactments of the human relationship to nature. Women in the menstrual hut submitted to the inevitable buildup of blood and its shedding. They passed through the underworld where natural forces preside. Every month they paid homage through ritual to the powers that sustain fragile human life. By this ritual act, the women held their human groups in relationship to the dark force which pulls the strings of chaos and disaster. Grahn argues convincingly that the mystery of menstruation was the motivation for the original creation of ritual. These menstrual rituals then spawned other rituals whose purpose was to transmit the meaning of the relationship between human beings and nature. Thus cultures began.

Women no longer perform this mediating role, no longer consciously carry, by means of a repeated ritual, the opposites of highly defined culture versus raw natural process. In modern life we are swept away by technical achievement which promises to overcome dark nature. In our exuberance, we lose sight of ourselves as animal beings at the mercy of a vast and intricate universe we barely comprehend. We lose our balanced standpoint which would include equally the fine achievements of culture along with the facts of our fated, fragile existence. In our imbalance, we have cut ourselves off from our roots as creatures of nature.

So unwieldy and heavily determined is modern culture that the only chance to realign with nature rests on the individual. The shedding of the demands of culture in order to encounter one's essential nature involves self-examination, self-exploration, and leads inescapably into the unconscious. Jung's psychology gives the individual the tools to explore the far reaches of the psyche, which after all is nature within the human being. To enter the gates of the unconscious is to step into an unknown realm where, at bottom, primordial nature resides. Descent in one sense is inevitable because as creatures within a culture, we are separated from the wilderness of our natural being. The psyche pulls us out of the confines of culture into a confrontation with our essential animal nakedness.

Much of the work of analysis involves shedding old adaptations that no longer fit the person's present-day life. The pain of this stripping comes when the person begins to face the real psychic injuries from the past which the false adaptation managed to obscure. The complex clinical understandings an analyst calls on to work with specific problems in analysis are not dealt with in this book. Rather, the subject here is the larger archetypal understructure that provides analyst and analysand a map or a matrix within which both are held while the intricate work of analysis takes place. The interaction between the archetypal matrix and the clinical particulars is the very stuff of analysis. That this book's main concern is the archetypal backdrop of the descent myth is not meant to imply that archetypal understanding can substitute for clinical expertise.

The archetypal pattern of descent, shedding the outdated structures of the psyche, is a long, arduous process. At times, it seems never ending, and indeed, remnants of our original psychic patterns maintain a hold all of our lives. Nevertheless, the psyche pulls for us to fall all the way to the bottom. At the bottom we meet ourselves stripped bare with nothing left but our mere existence. This condition of elemental reality burns into our consciousness. We return to the upper world bearing the imprint in our bones. The new carriers of the ancient watch on nature are these individuals who go all the way through a descent. The poet Enheduanna's lines describing devotees of Inanna fit the modern women who undergo descent:

those warrior women
like a single thread
come forth from beyond the river
do common work
in devotion to you
whose hands sear them with purifying fire
your many devoted
who will be burnt
like sun-scorched fire bricks
pass before your eyes

Inanna is said to cast over her devotees a net of lapis lazuli whose fine-eyed mesh traps them in her sway. Such a net is the descent myth, a jeweled matrix which sustains as it confines. Descent is built into the human psyche. Descent is an archetypal pattern none of us can avoid. Inanna's net confines us to our physical existence in matter. Yet it is made of deep blue lapis, the jewel most sacred to this goddess. When we finally understand that descent confers upon us the gift of our full individual, creative nature, placing us firmly in the reality of our circumstance on this planet, we can perhaps be more tolerant of the suffering the process demands. I invite you then to join me in the reorientation of attitude the descent myth requires as we undertake together to uncurse the dark.

Acknowledgments

The origin of this book began with the childhood awakening in me of a religious sense, and I now recognize this great gift from my parents, Eva Harrell and Ralph De Shong. Ronnie Duggar kindly published my first piece in *The Texas Observer* thirty years ago. My friends at the C. G. Jung Institute of Los Angeles inspired me to write and gave me a space for intellectual and soul development. Thanks especially to the late Malcolm Dana, the late Hilde Kirsch, and to Janet Dallett. Thanks to Anne Kilmer for her support and for connecting me with Daniel A. Foxvog, who spent endless hours translating the descent myth and teaching me about the Sumerians and the Ancient Near East. I found in Judy Grahn a mentor who could help ground my intuitive ideas of women's development. To all the women who accompanied me under Judy's tutelage, especially Nisa Donnally and Kris Brandenburger, thanks for your support. The San Francisco Jung Institute offered a forum for Inanna and Enheduanna, and Elizabeth Osterman guided and supported me there with loving care. Mel Kettner was able to endure the rough ride through the underworld and remain a constant source of encouagement and love. Grateful thanks to Murray Stein, who suggested that I pull these essays together into a book, and to Siobhan Drummond, editor at Chiron Publications, who understood it all the first time and offered her creative attention and invaluable help.

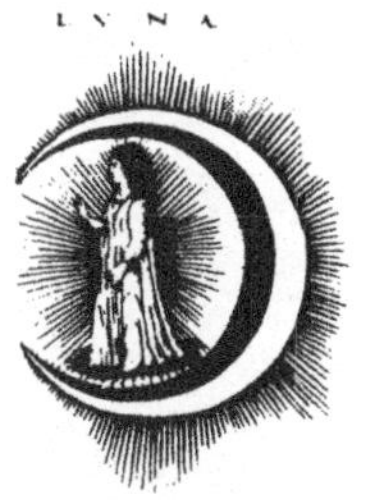

SECTION I
Blessingway

Blessingway Revisited

In the spring of 1963, I drove with my friends, Ruth and Bob Roessel, to Ruth's home on the Navajo reservation where she was to be the "one-sung-over" (Mitchell 1978, p. 3) in a Blessingway ritual. This was not my first visit to the Navajo with the Roessels. They had introduced me to that sparsely settled land of stark red buttes and had guided me through squaw dances in the summer and parts of the nine-night sings in the winter. During these rituals I had stood among the large surrounding crowd gathered to observe what an outsider was allowed to see.

On this occasion I was invited into the intimate circle of Ruth's family as a participant. I would be one of the ten to fifteen people sitting around the edge of the hogan watching the medicine man, Ruth's father, chant over her the ritual central to Navajo life, Blessingway. For three days and two nights, all of us would live, eat, and sleep inside the hogan, held in the matrix of Blessingway's sacred text and song.

At that time I was in my early thirties, the mother of three small children and a kindergarten teacher on the Salt River Indian Reservation near Phoenix. Four years before, I had left what now seems my tribal, provincial homeland in north Texas and left as well its central organizing institution, the Protestant church. These visits to the Navajo had a compelling attraction I barely understood. I knew nothing of the language, very little of the mythology and religion, but I found myself strangely drawn to Navajo life: the women corralling sheep or cooking fry bread or spinning and weaving; a Navajo couple on the seat of a horse-drawn wagon, silently enduring the slow, even pace of their ride.

Looking back thirty years I recognize what compelled me among the Navajo. In spite of the powerful influence of Western civilization surrounding the reservation, the Navajo way of life remains immersed in and oriented by the forces of nature. Life moves with the cycles of the seasons in an unending round.

The emphasis on harmony within the cycles of nature gives particular importance to women. *Kinaaldá*, the girl's menstruation ritual, is a key element in the life cycle of women and one of the gifts of Blessingway. The culture is matrifocal; married daughters continue to live near the homes of their mothers while sons move away to their wives' mothers' places. The revered female deity, Changing Woman, is central to Navajo religion. Having grown up in Texas with its image of manly bravado pervading every part of life, I had never imagined a culture which revolved around women, both in its economic life of sheep herding, corn growing, and weaving and in its mythology in which a goddess, Changing Woman, is the bounteous deity. During these visits, I had a small taste of being held and supported by a culture whose matrix is formed in large part out of the biological and instinctual experience of being female. For the first time, I was able to imagine living in a multifaceted culture that matched and respected my own female sensibilities, desires, needs, and major life changes from birth to death.

The central ritual of the Navajo, Blessingway, recites the story of Changing Woman. It tells of her birth, of her acquiring the sacred mountain soil bundle from her parents, First Man and First Woman; it tells that this "quiet little bundle" (Wyman 1970, p. 21) is to be in control of Blessingway, and that Blessingway is Changing Woman's own ceremonial. It tells of the construction of the first hogan where the hogan songs originated and where plans were being made for endowing natural phenomena with their inner forms. It says that beauty radiates from the inner spaces of the hogan. It tells that Changing Woman created people from the epidermal waste rubbed from her body. It recites the ritual observed at Changing Woman's first menstruation and her second menstruation, a ritual observed to this day by Navajo young women at the onset of puberty. It tells of Changing Woman's marriage, her children, her leaving to go to her home in the West. It gives instructions for the use of sacred pollen, for the cultivation of corn from planting to harvest. Changing Woman says, "Ever since I began to exist I have been right here among you. I shall continue to be everywhere. Whatever you are saying, I shall hear it all, my children" (ibid., p. 185). She says, "Every day, every night, every dawn, every year, your mother (Changing Woman) will be instructing you, but not by coming before you (in person). Arise, go to sleep, eat, drink, defecate, urinate, by means of all of these she will be instructing you" (ibid., p. 325).

Blessingway belongs to Changing Woman. At the core of it is the enlivening of the material world with divine inner forms. In Slim Curly's version of the Blessingway ritual, he speaks of the Holy People:

> "Now the purpose of placing these persons here is to have them become the inner forms of various things. After they have taken position at their interiors all of you will stand in position along the surface of this one called Earth Woman, you will pray to her, you will show her your respect. You will say my mother to her, you will say my grandmother to her," was said. (Wyman 1970, p. 123)

In Navajo religion, the live personalities of the inner forms, the Holy People, infuse all phenomena. "By themselves natural phenomena are lifeless, but an inner human form set within them functions as their life principle. This vitalizes and also personalizes each phenomenon" (Wyman 1970, pp. 23, 24). The divine substance not only is in matter but is in some way human. This human personality has the characteristics of a mother, of a grandmother. When you say to her "my mother," when you say to her "my grandmother," she responds to you, "my child." She is a divine being with the feelings of a human mother.

Earth Woman has a mate in the sky. Slim Curly says:

> You see, the one who became the inner form of earth, being a woman, was given charge of the care of things on earth and upward. On the upper side he who became inner form of sky, being a man, was charged with the care of things from above downward and the two themselves laid this down as a rule for themselves. (Wyman 1970, p. 133)

This divine pair hold the Navajo between them according to the rule of *Są'an naaghéi, Bik'eh hózhǫ́ǫ́*, "life constantly restored, according to which, conditions all around are blessed or made beautiful" (Mitchell 1980, p. 190). "Life constantly restored" intimates a constant, energetic force at work moving all life toward a harmonious condition of blessedness and beauty. The phrase implies a "condition" of natural phenomena that is continually reached but also continually fades in repetitive cycles and must be restored again, restored either by the natural cyclic process or by means of ritual such as Blessingway.

The Navajo religion anchors the people, *Diné*, solidly in the natural world. The divine beings, the Holy People, live inside natural phenomena and actively participate and interact with the people to restore life to its blessed condition. The Navajo religion positions itself firmly in matter where its divine beings live and thus is a religion based on the feminine principle of matter incarnate with the divine substance. Gods of the religions based on the masculine principle exist wholly outside nature in the world of spirit. While the Navajo religion is polytheistic and has both female and male gods, its central deity is female, Changing Woman.

Simply try to imagine interacting with plants, animals, stones, mountains, seeking each one's divine essence. Imagine immersing yourself in the natural world as one creature among billions, no one superior to the others. The demands of civilization so separate us from an attitude of respect for natural phenomena that it is difficult to return to or even approach such a perspective. Our huge Western egos strongly resist the diminishing necessary to walk among the Holy People in rocks, trees, wild animals.

The following essay, "A Blessingway Sing," contains all I could understand of the ritual at the time. I did not fathom that the compelling draw the Navajo had for me were the first stirrings of a long search for my roots as a woman in a religion based on the archetypal feminine premise that the divine infuses nature with her substance. All the essays in this book derive from the power of that compelling search. The Blessingway among the Navajo was the beginning.

A Blessingway Sing

Tempe, Ariz.

Happily, may I walk.
Happily, with abundant showers,
  may I walk.
Happily, with abundant plants,
  may I walk.
May it be beautiful before me.
May it be beautiful behind me.
May it be beautiful below me.
May it be beautiful above me.
May it be beautiful all around me.
In beauty it is finished.

from "The Night Chant"
(*Washington Matthews translation*)

If you go by way of Holbrook, you enter the Navajo reser-vation off Highway 66, a long trail west crowded with moving vans and displaced persons who think they'll find Life and a piece of the golden pot in California. The land is flat and grassy with a grey, brushy hill every once in a while or a mesa eroding dirty orange. Every couple of miles you see a hogan off in the distance with smoke rising out of the center hole. Hogans are built of logs and mud or sometimes plaster or even cinder block, but always facing east so that when you walk out early in the morning, the glaring Arizona sun hits you right in the face.

We were traveling to Round Rock, a small community consisting of a trading post, a Bureau of Indian Affairs school, a water tower, and hogans scattered for miles around. Four of us were in the cab of a pickup with a camper swaying like an elephant behind us: myself, my friends Ruth Roessel and her husband Bob, and their son, whom his father tenderly called "Little Indian Leader." He's three. Ruth was to be the patient in a Blessingway sing.

From *The Texas Observer*, January 24, 1964. Reprinted by permission.

It is a long drive from Phoenix to Round Rock, long even after you get on the reservation, which is the size of West Virginia. Near Round Rock, after climbing the "Big Red Hill," we picked out from the other grey lumps on the landscape the six or eight hogans that make up Ruth's home place, the homes of her sisters and their families and her mother and father. We pulled up beside her parents' hogan. Children and dogs scattered, both barking the news loudly.

I saw the swish of her mother's long skirt as she ducked inside the hogan. She had seen us but according to custom waited inside. We dawdled around the truck awhile, then walked in. The close relatives embraced, murmuring tenderly in Navajo. As they separated, we noted the changes in the interior of the hogan and exclaimed mildly in our adopted Navajo fashion. Ruth's parents had covered the dirt floor with cement and the walls with white beaver board. I guessed this had been done for the occasion. For the same reason, sheets covered the clothes hanging from hooks on the walls, and some of the pots and pans, a mattress, a trunk, and several sheepskins had been taken outside and set beside a bright yeibichai rug Ruth's mother was weaving under a ramada. She is well known as an excellent weaver.

As it grew dark, we put our blankets on the hogan floor and spread out a cold supper. One by one Ruth's sisters and brothers came in, the women in long skirts and velvet blouses, the men in western shirts and pants. Ruth had gifts for each of them, which they accepted with surprise and opened enthusiastically. They sat near the wall opposite us. Their several children crawled over the stretched-out legs of the men and through conversations of women on their haunches, evoking mild rebuffs. There was much gentle laughter.

Ruth's father signaled the beginning of the ceremony by raising himself up off the sheepskin where he'd been lying. A noted medicine man, he would perform the ceremony. He began taking objects out of his medicine man's pouch and placing them carefully on a square of white cloth on the floor near the wall opposite the door. Ruth was sitting on one side of these ceremonial objects and her father on the other. She had dressed in a white satin tiered skirt with a turquoise velvet overblouse and wore her prettiest turquoise and coral jewelry. She sat on a mattress covered with a large buffalo rug. Her father also had put on thick turquoise bracelets and a necklace and had tied a handkerchief around his forehead through his thick, shoulder length hair. The rest of us settled ourselves comfortably on blankets and sheepskins on one side of the hogan.

The Blessingway is a two-night sing and, says the late Father

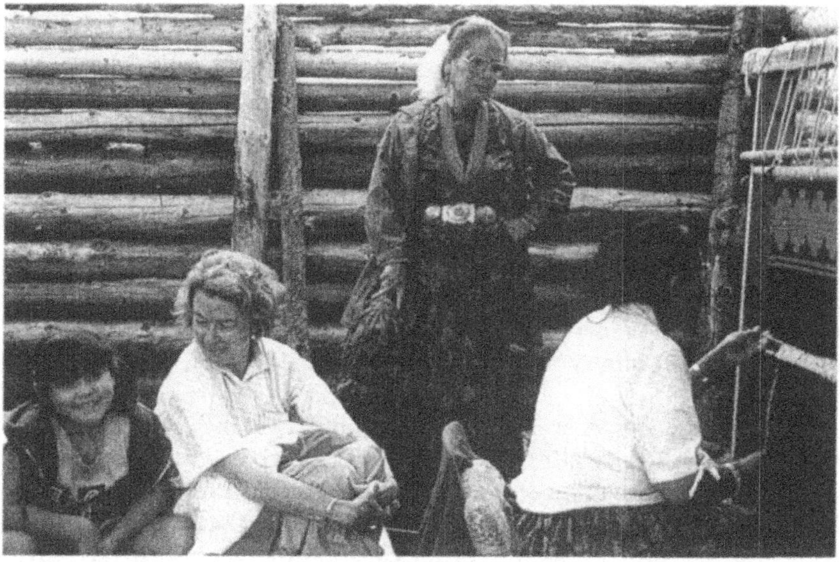

Figure 1. Ruth Roessel's sister Irene Tsinnijinnie, weaving, with Ruth (standing), Betty Meador, and Ruth's granddaughter Jaclyn Roessel (August 1990).

Berard Haile, "governs the entire Chantway system," which consists of thirty-five major ceremonials. Blessingway is addressed to the universe and invokes the powers of the universe that restore happiness, well-being, and harmony to the patient and, secondarily, the other participants in the sing. This first night, the medicine man seeks to drive away all the evil that may be in the hogan and all the evil that has caused disharmony in the patient. The patient's trouble is always determined beforehand by a diagnostician, and the ceremony prescribed is related to the illness. In this case, Ruth simply "didn't feel so good." Her father, some weeks before, had acted as diagnostician and prescribed Blessingway.

A coal oil lamp stood in its place in the center of the floor. Maiisani, Ruth's mother, enclosed its flue with a torn paper sack, and the light from it barely enabled us to see.

The medicine man began to sing the song prayers in Navajo. He stood and placed corn pollen on ceremonially prescribed parts of Ruth's body and passed the pollen pouch, made of unwounded deer skin, to Ruth's mother, who administered pollen to herself. We all did this then, each of us finishing by scattering a pinch of pollen from about chin level, moving the hand upward and out. This symbolizes the exit of evil.

This first night's ceremony took, I'd guess, a couple of hours. The patient and the medicine man moved from one side of the hogan to the other, and during most of the rest of the ceremony Ruth very rapidly repeated prayers that her father first said. She seemed to echo him, so quickly did she follow. The ceremony ended with more songs.

We sighed pleasurably when we stood and stretched, and we said goodnight softly to those who were leaving. We who were staying unfolded our bedrolls and with a minimum of conversation made ready for bed. We slept soundly all night on the hogan floor with our feet toward the squatty black wood stove in the center.

I lay in my sleeping bag a while after waking, contemplating the difficulty of extricating myself from this cocoon and enjoying the quiet drama on the other side of the room, illuminated by the coal oil lamp. Maiisani was preparing breakfast, stoking the fire, putting the coffee on, spreading a square of oil cloth on the floor near the stove on which she set cups and eating utensils. Ashishie (grandfather) raised himself out of his bed of sheepskin, from which he had seemed to be gently commanding the situation like a sultan. The family gathered around the food now waiting on the oil cloth, drank their thick, steaming coffee, and dipped hunks of bread into a pot of pork and beans. Two of the grandchildren had slept here, and both sat as close to Ashishie as they could, the younger accepting bites of bread from his grandfather's fingers.

This morning Ruth was to take the ceremonial bath, and after breakfast her father went out alone to find a proper yucca root that sudses like soap, while her mother prepared a small Navajo basket by pouring boiling water over it until its strands swelled tight.

Maiisani, who had assisted her husband the night before, now signaled the beginning of this portion of the ceremony by rubbing corn pollen near the roof at the four cardinal points of the hogan. The door was open, and the sun managed to get around and under an army blanket nailed over the opening that told passersby a ceremony was going on inside. Ruth had taken her hair down out of the butterfly knot Navajos wear and had taken off her blouse in the old Navajo way. A young girl stifled a snicker.

Maiisani crossed the water-filled basket with corn pollen. It lay a few feet from the other ceremonial objects. Ashishie began to sing. At the appointed time, Ruth washed her hair with the yucca suds, using the water in the basket. Several of the women held up blankets to shield Ruth as she completed her bath amid giggles and exclamations about the coldness of the water. Ashishie sang more prayer songs after the bath and the ceremony concluded.

The rest of the morning, each of us who were participating knelt before the water basket and washed our hair, sudsing in our palms the fraying yucca root. The families casually took turns, the women heating more water, their long hair falling over their shoulders down to their waists, the children reluctantly yielding to their mother's coaxing, bending over the small basket: we all washed ourselves.

Ruth was not to do any sort of work during the ceremony and set the tone for the rest of us. We spent the afternoon lazily wandering, or halfheartedly doing the chores which had to be done, or contemplating the surrounding mountains and buttes. The Lukachuki Mountains and Sleeping Lady, who lies on top of them, stretched across the eastern horizon. Jutting out from the mountains are great red cliffs; against the deep blue mountains they are like docks against a harbor. To the Navajo these mountains are sacred, and like all things sacred to them, they have a "real" name unknown to most outsiders. This name identifies the "soul" of the mountain or that mystery the Navajo experiences in relationship with the mountains. Persons who come to know each other in a deep closeness are said to know each other's real name, or in an experience of the mystery or awesomeness of a part of nature a Navajo learns its real name. I am reminded of once hearing W. H. Auden say that in a poem the poet tries to give the real name to a sacred (awe-inspiring) experience.

Two of the sisters had killed a sheep in the afternoon, and we had lamb stew and cabrito for supper, along with a delicious dried, then soaked corn bread. The night's ceremony was to last until dawn; we all went to sleep about nine.

One by one we followed Ashishie's slow waking movements around one o'clock. Maiisani spread a blanket in front of her daughter and husband, and we all placed on it objects to be blessed. Most of us, according to tradition, put forward only our shoes, but others piled on top of them baskets, jewelry, purses, a harness, clothes. Maiisani sprinkled corn pollen on each object to begin the ceremony.

We sat in a semicircle, with Ruth and her father at the top of the arch we made. Most of the children were awake and sat staring big-eyed into the paper-covered lamp. Those who knew them began to sing joyously the hogan songs. They are strong courageous songs of blessing and assurance. Ashishie shifted himself at the end of the song group, spat into a tin can, and lit a cigarette. The others of us relaxed and talked quietly.

The second group of songs began, and so, on until dawn, we followed this pattern of songs and pause, intermittently passing the buckskin bag of pollen around the semicircle, careful not to miss anyone and sprinkling pollen on those who had dropped off to sleep. Toward dawn, the singers seemed to challenge the first rays, knowing they would soon appear, voicing a confidence and joy as strong as any sun that ever shone.

The patient was now an empty vessel. In anxious silence the medicine man made a trail of pollen from his seat to the door. The patient rose and walked on the path out the door into a grey-silver world. There, alone, she would breathe in new life from the sun. The ceremony was over.

Driving home I was conscious of my blessed shoes: now I would walk in beauty. I wondered how much of the Navajo's renewal of life and harmony from these ceremonies grows out of a superstition that godlike forces acted upon them; or how much of it comes from a consciousness that they could, and indeed must if it can be found, themselves choose the way of beauty, of which the ceremony is a symbolic structured vessel. Or how many combinations of such possibilities there were. Or if it really makes any difference when new courage and joy are the result.

I viewed the signs of "civilization" with a certain sadness. Such an unwieldy way of life we lead. Where is our healing in this neon maze?

Some weeks later, at a conference for Indian leaders, I overheard Bob and Ruth Roessel talking to Karl Menninger, who has been closely associated with various Indian groups for thirty years. Ashishie was to be the patient in a ceremony which Dr. and Mrs. Menninger would attend.

"You see," said Bob, "a medicine man uses all of his resources in healing. He becomes depleted. He has to have a sing in order to be restored." The famous Dr. Menninger bent from the waist in an attitude of humility. "Oh I know. I know," he said. "That's why I'm out here."

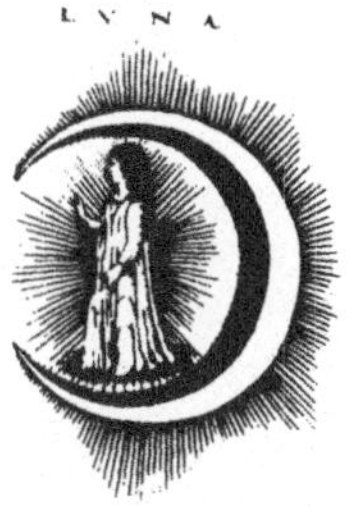

SECTION II
The Seven Gates

The Stripping

The essays in this book represent a search for a time when the imagination of women could be nourished in a female atmosphere that allows creative works to flourish. The belief which fostered the essays is that a female imagination, an imagination born out of the biological experience of being a woman, is a part of the basic structure of every woman's psyche. Because the expressions of the female imagination remain largely hidden, repressed in the dark of the unconscious, superseded by the predominant masculine imagination which has created and ordered Euro-American culture, those expressions require an active search on the part of the individual woman. The title, *Uncursing the Dark,* is shorthand for the activity of that search.

I do not condemn male-imagined culture. Rather, I grieve the lack, the loss, the absence of a concomitant female-imagined culture which could flourish side-by-side, if only there were breathing room. I grieve the stunted and distorted lives of women who, shaped by the imperatives of the masculine imagination, abort the embryos of their own creativity long before gestation has completed its natural cycle.

I am not talking about imposing "femaleness" on little girls. Quite the opposite. I am starting from the premise that girls and women necessarily, because of their sex, have the innate propensity to experience and perceive the world from a different slant. In Jung's terms, that slant would issue from the archetypal feminine which hovers close to a woman's experience of herself. At bottom the archetypal feminine is the imagination of female instinctuality, the imagination stirred by her biological femaleness. Let her imagination thrive in a culture-free zone. What would she create? Allow her freedom to soar in a culture that prizes the work of women. Who would she become? Raise her in a male-imagined culture where her sex, her slant, is excluded at best, disparaged at worst, she adapts to the cultural imperatives for survival's sake.

What stirred me on those visits to the Navajo reservation were the women. Something in what I saw, the communal life, the women gently shaping the order of the day, corralling the sheep, herding the sheep, sitting on the ground spinning wool, weaving rugs, grinding corn, preparing the ritual basket, washing their long hair, something touched off a reverberating chord, awakened a sensibility already present. I felt that I was home, that I had only been away for a while in a foreign country. The women of the Navajo, I now see, live in a culture that honors and makes room for female imagination.

Get beyond the belief that I romanticize the Navajo. I do not romanticize the dirt hardness of life on the reservation. Focus on this experience: a culture whose people organize their lives around the sensibilities of a female imagination (as well as male) touched a familiar chord in this woman, sparked a recognition in herself of an innate configuration of femaleness which lay dormant beneath an adaptation to her own culture.

The world of Euro-American women has changed considerably since that trip to the Navajo reservation in 1963. In spite of the changes and the increased consciousness of women, any individual woman still has to become aware of the restrictions that the culture imposes on her lively, natural self. The first step toward retrieval of her female imagination involves a stripping of elements of the thwarting adaptation she has made.

Two pieces follow, a portion of the myth "Inanna's Descent to the Underworld" and an essay, "Doris Lessing's Apocalyptic Vision." Each discloses that painful, essential first step a woman has to take toward a retrieval of the female imagination. The woman has to be stripped bare of the trappings her culture has imposed over her natural self. The task is, of course, impossible. She cannot strip herself of the intricate web of cultural imperatives within which she lives.

Inanna could do that because she is a goddess. Doris Lessing's heroine could do that because she lives solely in the imagination. Our real live woman can only approach this thorough stripping. The descent myth and Lessing's novel show us the way, give us the courage an example affords. As myths, the one ancient, the other modern, they present a pattern, an archetypal instance of a terrible downgoing. They exemplify the necessary shedding of outmoded, inappropriate adaptations that hinder access to the feminine Self.

The myth, "Inanna's Descent to the Underworld," originates in ancient Mesopotamia, 3500 B.C. or before. In the myth, Inanna, the bright goddess of the upper world, the star we call Venus, the epitome of the fine achievements of the Sumerian civilization, decides on her own to go to the underworld realm where her older sister, Ereshkigal, reigns. Consider Inanna. She is queen of heaven and earth. She is the predominant goddess in a culture that thrives on its inventions–the wheel, the written word–and on its achievements–world trade, architectural grandeur, teeming cities, political order, ritual concordance. The beginning lines of the myth say that Inanna, from her position in the highest heaven, turned her ear toward the great below. Inanna heard something or listened for something. Whatever she heard determined her decision to go to the underworld. I imagine she recognized a lack, a missing sensibility, a content, an experience, an understanding she, in all her brilliant representation of human achievement, did not have. That something could be found in the underground world of her older sister, Ereshkigal.

The myth carries a double message. One is that the accomplishments of civilization based on the masculine imagination (as the Sumerian civilization was by this time, having invented kings, weapons, armies, hierarchies) focuses on achievement, and that focus separates its citizens from an ongoing awareness of primordial nature. Inanna sought to bridge that separation by directing her consciousness toward the primordial dark of the underworld.

The other message of the myth is that primordial nature is ruled by a female, a goddess, Ereshkigal. Inanna, who has so successfully adapted to Sumerian civilization, ruling from her position of queen of the upper world, has lost her connection to the vast feminine world of natural processes, natural cycles.

Male-imagined culture separates us as women from our harmonious concordance with nature. Our bodies bleed with the moon. Our bodies harbor the gestating child. We are biologically attuned to instinct's dark realm. Unless we retrieve that connection consciously, we wander half-alive in someone else's skin. That retrieval depends on our ability to translate from body to psyche, from an awareness of actual cycle and periodicity to the dark intuitive language of the imaginal. Ereshkigal, queen of this underworld realm, pulls us monthly into her bloody corridors. Her gifts lie behind every door.

Come then. With your rich fantasy, follow Inanna into the underworld.

The Descent of Inanna to the Underworld

The Seven Gates

I

	in great heaven
SHE	turned her ear
	to great earth
	in great heaven
THE GODDESS	turned her ear
	to great earth
	in great heaven
INANNA	turned her ear
	to great earth
	left heaven
MY LADY	abandoned earth
	went down below
	left heaven
INANNA	abandoned earth
	went down below
	where she ruled the city
	she left
	where she ruled the temple
	she left

This rendition of the descent myth is by Betty Meador with the translation and assistance of Dr. Daniel Foxvog.

SHE WENT DOWN BELOW

she left Uruk
    temple of An
    Eanna
she went down below

she left Badtibira
    halo of the land
    Emushkalamma
she went down below

she left Zabalam
    sky terrace temple
    Giguna
she went down below

she left Adaba
    measured gardens
    Esharra
she went down below

she left Nippur
    temple of the throne
    Baradurgarra
she went down below

she left Kish
    temple of the mountains
    Hursagkalamma
she went down below

she left Agade
    little flower temple
    Eulmash
she went down below

seven sacred powers bound to her side
sacred powers gathered in her hand
sacred powers firm under foot
she left

she wound a crown of pure cloth
crown of the wild steppe
on her head
a beauty shone through hair locks on her brow

she held the lapis measuring reed
and coiled the royal field rope in her hands

at her neck she tied lapis beads
twin egg stones filled her breast

gold ring on her hand
breast plate *man-come-come*
she wrapped herself in royal robes
the perfume *may-he-come* trailed after her glance

INANNA WENT DOWN BELOW

II

Ninshubur
Chosen Lady
follows

pure Inanna
calls her

my rock
faithful mistress of Eanna
good-word-bearer
carrier of true words
COME

I am going down below
when I reach that place
    wail for me
    cry in lamentation by the ruins
    play a drum song
    drum for me in the throne court
    wander for me
    wander through the houses of the gods

    tear at your eyes
    tear at your mouth
    tear at the place you show no one

    wear rags for me
    only rags

then
set your feet towards Enlil's house
go alone to Enlil's house
    Great Mountain Temple
    Ekur
enter Enlil's great mountain house
look him in the eye and
WEEP

say
    father Enlil
    do not let anyone
    hold your daughter down
    below

    do not let your
    good silver
    mix with the dust of that place

    do not let your
    precious lapis lazuli
    be split with the mason's stone

do not let your
sweet boxwood
be sawn with the carpenter's wood

do not let the maiden
Inanna
be held down below
if Enlil does not help you
go to Ur

In Ur
Nanna's temple
Moon God Temple
House-of-Light
Ekishnugal
go to Nanna
look him in the eye and
WEEP

say
father Nanna
do not let anyone
hold your daughter down below

do not let your
good silver
mix with the dust of that place

do not let your
precious lapis lazuli
be split with the mason's stone

do not let your
sweet boxwood
be sawn with the carpenter's wood

do not let the maiden
Inanna
be held down below
if Nanna does not help you
go to Eridu

In Eridu
enter the temple of Enki
look him in the eye and
WEEP

say
father Enki
do not let anyone
hold your daughter down below

do not let your
good silver
mix with the dust of that place

do not let your
precious lapis lazuli
be split with the mason's stone

do not let your
sweet boxwood
be sawn with the carpenter's wood

do not let the maiden
Inanna
be held down below

wise father Enki
lord of wide ear
  who knows the life-giving plant
  who knows the life-giving water
he is the one
to restore me
to life

I go
Ninshubur
do not follow

go Ninshubur
do what I say
do not forsake
the word I speak

III

Inanna
  at Ganzir
  netherworld gate

Inanna
  pushing
  netherworld gate

Inanna
  cries out
  at netherworld gate

Open UP
Doorman
Open Up the House

I am alone
LET ME IN

Open UP
Neti
Open Up the House

I am alone
LET ME IN

Neti
        great doorman
        of the netherworld
Neti answers
pure Inanna
        YOU
        who are you?

I am Inanna
star of evening
traveling toward the dawn

YOU
Inanna
star of evening
traveling toward the dawn
        why are you here
        in the land-of-no-return?
        what led your heart
        where no traveler turns back?

pure Ereshkigal
my older sister
for her I have come

her lord
Gugalanna
has died

the Great Bull of Heaven
has died

I have come for his funeral
take part in his wake is why I have come

Neti
        great doorman
        of the netherworld
Neti answers
pure Inanna

stand there
Inanna
I must speak to my queen
I must speak to Ereshkigal
tell her what you say

Neti
        great doorman
        of the netherworld
Neti enters
the house of his queen

MY QUEEN
Ereshkigal
a maiden alone stands outside
your sister Inanna
has come to Ganzir
she pushed at the door
cried out at the gate

she left Eanna temple
to come down below

seven sacred powers bound to her side
sacred powers gathered in her hand
sacred powers firm under foot
she comes

she wound a crown of pure cloth
crown of the wild steppe
on her head
a beauty shines through hair locks on her brow

she holds the lapis measuring reed
and coils the royal field rope in her hands

at her neck she ties lapis beads
twin egg stones fill her breast

gold ring on her hand
breast plate *man-come-come*
she wraps herself in royal robes
the perfume *may-he-come* trails after her glance

INANNA IS HERE BELOW

Ereshkigal
slaps her thighs
bites her lips

says
    Neti
    great doorman of the netherworld
    come here
    listen
    do exactly what I say

    bolt the seven gates of the netherworld
    then
    one by one
    open each door
    open each door
    of the Palace Ganzir

let her come in
capture her
strip off her clothes
carry them away
bring her to me

Neti
great doorman of the netherworld
obeys the word of his queen

he fastens the bolts
of the seven gates

one by one
he opens each door
of the Palace Ganzir

he says out loud
    COME
    INANNA
    ENTER

when Inanna comes in
someone takes from her head
the crown of pure cloth

    WHAT IS THIS

silent Inanna
sacred customs
must be fulfilled
do not open your mouth
against this rite

when she enters the second gate
someone takes from her neck
the lapis beads

WHAT IS THIS

silent Inanna
sacred customs
must be fulfilled
do not open your mouth
against this rite

when she enters the third gate
someone removes
twin egg stones from her royal breast

WHAT IS THIS

silent Inanna
sacred customs
must be fulfilled
do not open your mouth
against this rite

when she enters the fourth gate
someone removes
the breast plate *man-come-come*

WHAT IS THIS

silent Inanna
sacred customs
must be fulfilled
do not open your mouth
against this rite

when she enters the fifth gate
someone removes
the gold ring from her hand

WHAT IS THIS

silent Inanna
sacred customs
must be fulfilled
do not open your mouth
against this rite

when she enters the sixth gate
someone takes from her hand
the coiled measuring line of lapis

WHAT IS THIS

silent Inanna
sacred customs must be fulfilled
do not open your mouth
against this rite

when she enters the seventh gate
someone unwraps
the Lady's royal robe
someone strips away
the Ladyship royal robe

she is naked now and bowed low

WHAT IS THIS

silent Inanna
sacred customs
must be fulfilled
do not open your mouth
against this rite

Doris Lessing's Apocalyptic Vision

Of all the world religions, only Judaism, Christianity, and Islam have no feminine figure in the godhead. All other religions around which a people has been centered, from the earliest stone statues of 30,000 B.C., through the dawn of civilization in the Middle East to the Greeks, including the historical primitive religions and those still existing, all have varieties of images of the goddess.

We surmise that the disappearance of the goddess in Judaism, Christianity, and Islam was related to a major development in the history of consciousness. Around 1000 B.C. there appears to have been a great archetypal masculine thrust responding to the need to coagulate and expand the fragile, emerging logos and rationality of humankind. The pull of the Mother Goddess toward the Earth was compensated by a soaring of the spirit into the masculine realm, and in the three religions born of this development the goddess was nowhere seen. Her presence not being manifest, she was thus underground, concealed in the unconscious. She appeared briefly among the Gnostics, who spoke of a divine Mother, but this sect was ruled heretical by the Catholic fathers.

Jung has made available to our understanding of the workings of the psyche the rule of opposites. If one pole of an opposite is dominant and thus in consciousness, the other pole lives and builds and works in the unconscious. Thus during the 3,000 years of conscious dominance in the Western world of a masculine god, a concomitantly powerful feminine presence has been building in the unconscious. In his book *Aion*, Jung predicted that the present age would see a reemergence of the archetypal feminine into consciousness. The goddess in her various forms, who has been obscured in the unconscious, will begin to erupt into the conscious world.

If Jung's prediction that we can expect a resurgence of the archetype of the feminine is correct, we should be able to see the effects

---

across a broad spectrum. This is indeed the case. For two decades the women's movement has had an increasingly widespread appeal, and its effect on the social status of women is well known. The Amazon image of the goddess seems to dominate here. In the United States as well as other countries, a renewed focus on ecology seems inspired by the fecund, nourishing mother image of the feminine. The increasing awareness of healthful and harmful foods as well as therapies which focus on manipulation of the body to heal psychological disturbances suggest a new appreciation of the physical body, the concrete matter of our human existence, our unavoidable relationship to the Mother. Even the new morality, to the extent that multiple sexual relationships are an accepted part of women's lives, suggests a release of the Aphrodite image into drawing rooms where her presence has never been allowed.

All of these concerns involve groups of people and come under the aegis of sociology, but what of the individual woman into whose unsuspecting life the archetype of the feminine erupts, challenging the traditional model she had been following? Certainly if there is a general emergence of the archetype, it will be seen not only sociologically but will be felt as an upheaval by individuals as well.

The psychological disturbance that this situation can produce in an individual is the subject of several of Doris Lessing's novels. In *Summer Before the Dark*, the heroine, Kate, is living the traditional dream life. She is happily married to a successful surgeon, has three beautiful children, and is fulfilling her role as wife and mother. Unexpectedly, a new consciousness seeps into her awareness, a consciousness of her individuality as a woman which does not fit the role she is living. Kate endures the eruption of a psychosis in the process of reclaiming herself (Lessing 1973).

A series of novels whose heroine is named Martha Quest culminates in the book, *The Four-Gated City*. In this book, Martha realizes that a whole world of truth lies hidden from ordinary view in the inner world of the psychotic. Martha deliberately isolates herself in order to sink into the terror of her own unconscious and manages to traverse this underworld. She emerges with new psychic capacities which she and other initiates are able to use to communicate telepathically following a disaster that virtually destroys civilized life (Lessing 1969).

The most direct portrayal of the new presence of a goddess in the life of a woman is in Lessing's novel, *Memoirs of a Survivor*. The novel is an allegory whose heroine is coping with the gradual destruction of her world. I would like to look at this novel as an artist's intuitive vision of the effects of the emerging feminine.

The narrator of the novel is a middle-aged woman through whose eyes we watch the slow, painful disintegration of a city. The evolving disaster is of apocalyptic dimension, reminiscent of the disaster in *The Four-Gated City*. The beginning or cause for the disaster is cloaked in mystery. All public services are disrupted. The city administrators and law protectors cry with helpless voices against an erosion that spreads with a life of its own.

In Lessing's view, the enormity of the change is apocalyptic. The old ways will be destroyed. The rule of the patriarchy which has held civilization together will come down. We will experience chaos and anarchy. Applied to an individual, the disaster is shattering the woman's world. A force whose source she does not know and whose inevitability she comes to accept is slowly and persistently destroying everything that gave order, stability, and meaning to her life. She is experiencing an apocalypse within the boundary of her own psyche. The shift from a world dominated by the patriarchy to a more balanced masculine/feminine consciousness will not come gently, according to Lessing. The shift will bring a total disruption of civilized life on the outside and extreme psychic distress to the inner world of the individual.

The novel, then, is the story of one woman coping with such an apocalyptic inner event. We don't know her name; she is simply the narrator. As the story begins, she is looking back on the events which have happened. She recalls when her neighbors first became aware of "it." "It" seems to be an impersonal force, undefinable, "like a strange fish from the sea," she says, a force before which human understanding and adequacy is helplessly small. The survivors recall the ludicrous game all agreed to play in order to ignore the fact that "it" was dissolving the ground beneath their feet. "There is nothing people won't try to accommodate into ordinary life," she says. Finally, the disintegrating events preclude playing the game any longer. "It," as the force that was destroying their city, was brought into consciousness and given a name, if only "it."

The woman remembers that shortly after becoming aware of "it," she discovered, as she gazed at a particular spot on her living room wall when the morning light accented faded flowers on the wallpaper beneath a coat of paint, that the wall would dissolve and she could go through into an unknown space beyond. She realized she had been hearing sounds from behind the wall all of her life, and perhaps those sounds, that life behind the wall, was every bit as important as her ordinary life.

The woman had discovered the unconscious. It is no accident

that her beginning relationship to her inner life (the life behind the wall) coincided with her conscious acknowledgment of "it," the impersonal force that had invaded life in the outer world and was causing drastic changes. Such an eruption of the unconscious affects happenings in ordinary collective life as well as happenings in the psyches of individuals.

Behind the wall the woman finds rooms upon rooms, rooms which she intuits hold what she needs, what she has been waiting for all of her life. She feels there an awareness of a sweet Presence, the conviction of a promise, of reassurance. This ghostly Presence, she concludes, is the exiled rightful inhabitant of the rooms behind the wall.

Her first reaction is to escape. She wants either to leave the city to escape the disintegrating effects of "it" or to go behind the wall and stay there. She has become aware that the meaning which contained her life no longer holds. She either wants to escape to a place "it" hasn't touched or build up a wall against "it." Or she may try to hide in the unconscious, pull its sweet presence around her like a cloak and mask with the so-called spiritual life the grim necessity of facing reality.

Fortunately for this woman, fate intervenes with a task that keeps her exactly where she is. A strange man knocks on her door, shoves a preteenage girl into her apartment, and says, "Here, she's your responsibility." The woman is puzzled, runs after the man, but he has disappeared. The girl walks quietly into the room accompanied by her pet, an ugly animal that appears to be part dog and part cat. The woman accepts that she must keep the girl (Emily) and, given the strangeness of the other happenings around her, she soon stops questioning why.

Very soon we discover that behind the walls lives a family whose painful, stifling interactions the woman watches with feelings of smothering pressure. It is Emily's family, and the little girl being teased and lusted after by her officer father, then corrected, handled, and openly disparaged by her mother, is Emily herself. The puzzle of the story begins to unravel. The woman finds in the unconscious painful memories of childhood. She reexperiences these awful scenes and re-understands their impact on her life. The woman, then, is Emily, too, and the adolescent who appears at her door as her responsibility signifies the possibility of refinding the self buried in the child. "Had Emily been some kind of prisoner?" the woman asks herself at the beginning of their acquaintance. Yes, she had. She had been imprisoned in the expectations and old values learned from her father and mother. Now as the world crumbles, the prisoner is freed but painfully stripped of her identity.

The atmosphere in the world behind the wall in which the family appears is thick and heavy. This part of the world she calls the "personal." On other visits, she enters the world of the "impersonal." The impersonal world at first is characterized by an atmosphere of light and of possibility. She looks forward to her visits there with sweet anticipation. Later, as the number of visits increases, she discovers a change in the impersonal world. The rooms are in disarray. Chairs and tables are turned over. Curtains are pulled down, and the walls are spattered with filth. Dutifully she cleans and straightens and scrubs, but inevitably on her next visit to these same rooms, some trickster has whirled through and created a chaotic mess all over again. Again she scrubs and straightens and cleans and mends, and on and on in a seemingly endless task she sets things right in the rooms only to find them scattered again as soon as she turns around. With painstaking persistence the woman tackles the disarray in her unconscious. Just when she thinks she has faced and accepted what she finds, she turns to see the ordered rooms flung into chaos.

Finally, one day, she decides to paint the walls of a particular room. She scrubs, finds paint, and applies layer after layer. It is beautiful, "like standing inside a cleaned-out eggshell." She says, "I felt that accretions of grime had been taken off which had been preventing a living thing from breathing." After this, the trickster-destroyer stops his play, or rather, she never sees this room again. The unconscious shows its mercurial nature, its thousand eyes. Lessing's heroine says, "While I was in that room, the task made sense; there was continuity to what I did, a future, and I was in a continuing relation to the invisible destructive creature, or force, just as I was with the other beneficent presence. But this feeling of relatedness, of connection, of context, belonged to that particular visit to the room, and on the next visit it was not the same room, and my preoccupation with it was altered–and so with the other rooms, other scenes, whose flavors and scents held total authenticity for the time they lasted and not a moment longer."

In the midst of the woman's compelling new relationship to the unconscious sits the young girl, Emily, a heavy dose of reality. Their relationship is strained and polite. Emily is bursting into womanhood through every pore and just as powerfully restraining herself from action. The tension is almost unbearable. In the chaotic situation outside their apartment, gangs of young people have begun gathering into set groups, new communities. Emily and the woman watch these gangs on the corner across from their building. Emily, not yet brave enough to join the gangs on the pavement, stores up energy and tension in gluttony. She eats, sleeps, and bloats. Then suddenly, in an inexplicable turnaround, she begins to lose her excess and becomes consumed with finding an image through the clothes she wears. She tries on one costume after another until she finally breaks out into the world and shyly approaches the edge of the gangs on the pavement. The desperate insecurity of having no firm image of herself is overcome by the passion to be one like the others.

A difficulty develops in Emily's approach to the gangs. In the current shortage of food, dogs are not exempt from the diet. Emily watches horrified as the teenagers eye her precious Hugo. With the understanding of instinct, Hugo tries to hide behind his mistress. Emily grabs him just in time and returns him to the apartment.

In the weeks that follow, Emily becomes a part of a particular gang led by a strapping, idealistic adolescent named Gerald. Other gangs form, collect supplies, and move on, supposedly out of the city into safer places in the country. Emily's group, however, finds an empty house not far from the apartment and moves in. Emily becomes Gerald's number one woman. She falls in love with him and blossoms into womanhood with her initiation into sexuality.

Hugo, out of necessity, has to be left behind. He sits despondent with his nose poked through a slit in the drawn curtains or huddles far from the window when gang members taunt him from outside. Seen as a psychological symbol, Hugo is Emily's instinctual connection to her own precious, inborn uniqueness, and ultimately her connection to the transpersonal Self. It is said of Hugo that he has green cat eyes in an ugly dog's body. He is a strange beast. He, like the loathsome dwarf, holds the secret, the key, the pearl of great price beneath his ugly countenance. As an adolescent, she discards him in order to be like the others. Gang members stalk the apartment hoping for a chance to grab this delicate morsel. Individuality is dangerous to the life of the tribe. It has to be hidden away or discarded in favor of collective values.

The woman watches Emily with the patience of knowing the young woman must go through these experiences. She says she is waiting "for Emily to step off this merry-go-round, this escalator carrying her from the dark into the dark." Finally Emily becomes disenchanted with Gerald and returns home. Her disenchantment coincides with a new quality the woman experiences behind the wall. Earth has blown in, a forest, boundlessness, a new sense of the Presence, and personally the girl Emily experiences a lessening of the urgent sense of protest she'd always felt. Emily steps off the merry-go-round where she was wedded to the heroic attitude of conquering evil, an attitude of self-righteous protest. While this is a defeat for idealism, it opens new vistas in the inner world of the unconscious.

At this point, the woman is once again tempted to leave the city. She herself, for the first time, crosses the street to stand with the new gangs that are forming. Now the gangs typically include adults and old people along with the young. She is strongly tempted to give up her life and what's left of civilization and leave. She seeks an outer solution to replace the slow, tedious, painful work of facing herself. She looks for an easier way through drowning the demands of the unconscious with outer activity. Thoughts of the young Emily pull her back. She seems to know instinctively that sticking with the process of maturation is the only way she will rediscover her true self.

Her visits behind the wall are punctuated with the persistent cry of a baby. Even back in her apartment with Emily she hears the baby cry. Searching and searching for her, she finally discovers the child and to her surprise, it is not the baby Emily she had seen in so many other painful visits, but Emily's mother as a baby. The pattern of despair and unconscious neglect has repeated itself for who knows how many generations.

A further increment of disintegration outside is announced by the appearance of a new breed of children. There had been gangs of kids before, kids who had run away or been deserted by their parents. These new children are different. They behave as though they never had parents. They are completely uncivilized. They live underground in the sewers like moles or rats. The former gangs had rules. These children do not. The people call them wicked. Gerald is intent on containing them, hopefully civilizing them a bit. He comes to Emily and begs her to return to help him. She finally gives in. However, these new children prove too much for Gerald's organized household. Their amorality and destructiveness drive away the former members, and soon only Emily is left. Gerald takes the children away to more secure quarters. The woman finds Emily alone and persuades her to come home.

The adults who remain in her neighborhood are terrified of these children. They hover in their houses or apartments, afraid to go out. The air outside becomes more and more noxious. Water, if it is available, is no longer pure. Packs of dogs roam the streets tearing at any living animal. The woman wonders if she will be next. She is surrounded by a primitive anarchy which reeks of evil. A neighbor in a meeting suggests that they each take one of the new children in order to disperse their effect, but the children on hearing this bare their teeth and run away, wielding clubs, knives, and sticks.

The eruption of an amoral, evil force parallels a theme of a novel from the 1920s by Bruno Goetz, *A Kingdom Without Space* (1919). In it, gangs of boys roam the streets led by a Pied Piper-like figure named Fo. These boys are pitted against the light forces of goodness and Christianity which are icy cold, sterile and lifeless. Goetz apparently sensed that life had gone out of Christianity and that the reappearance of life would come through a Dionysian abandon with its dangerous frenzy and potential for evil. Dionysus is a god strongly connected to the Mother Goddess. The two opposite poles in Goetz's novel are hopelessly far apart and irreconcilable. Jung, on reading the Goetz novel, was struck by the similarity of the brown boys and the brown-shirted Nazi youth following Hitler.

Lessing's novel comes some fifty years after Goetz's. We have lived through the hideous eruption of evil which was Nazi Germany. Lessing offers a more hopeful conclusion and possibility for integration of the alien force these children represent by suggesting that an individual has to face and carry the evil of it within her or his psyche.

Gerald in our story finally gives up his dogged determination to change the children. He is shocked when little Denis, only four, kills an old man. (*Los Angeles Times*, July 18, 1980: teenage boys douse a four-year-old with gasoline and set him afire.) Gerald's final defeat comes when the children turn on him and begin to stone him. Emily, watching from the apartment, runs to rescue Gerald, who still can hardly believe what is happening. The adolescent hero is reluctant to give up the belief that his idealism can save the world.

What follows is a long period of waiting. Emily, Gerald, Hugo, and the woman huddle together in the apartment, terribly alone, barely managing to keep food and water and fuel. The world behind the wall has been silent for a long time, ever since the appearance of the new children. The woman last saw Emily there, as an adolescent in a vulgar red dress, writhing and contorting sexually before her mother's eyes.

One day, as winter finally passes, a yellow stain of sunlight appears on the wall, and it opens. The woman calls Emily and Gerald excitedly. They walk into that other world, the world "of a thousand little flashes, a jumble of little scenes." The woman watches; there stands Gerald, Emily, her officer father, "her large laughing gallant mother," and little Denis holding Gerald's hand. The group walks on, led by the One she had been looking for all this time, the sweet

Presence. She gets only a glimpse of her face "like the fading of a spark on dark air." Emily is there, "but quite beyond herself, transmuted, and in another key, and the yellow beast Hugo fitted her new self: a splendid animal, handsome, all kindly dignity and command, he walked beside her and her hand was on his neck." The One who went ahead "led them out of this collapsed little world into another order of world altogether." At the last moment Gerald turns and sees his children running excitedly after him, "clinging to his hands and his clothes, and they all followed quickly on after the others as the last walls dissolved."

This final scene is one of psychic integration and movement into a totally new level of consciousness. The events preceding are instructive. The last holdout, the hero animus, finally accepts his impotence against the evil, amoral condition of the children. The characters wait in poverty with no word from behind the wall. As in the dark night of the soul, God has forsaken them. Then, without warning, the unconscious opens in a scene of radiant transformation.

Seen psychologically, the woman has done her tedious, painful work. She has cleaned and recleaned the disordered rooms in her inner world. She has faced and accepted the sad truths of her childhood. She has patiently allowed her young self to grow into adulthood and suffered the indignity of her idealistic animus's defeat. Significantly, she even accepts little Denis, the murderer. She accepts not just her personal shadow, but the possibility of impersonal evil housed in her psyche. The effect of this work is a chiseling away at ego demands for grandeur, leaving her stripped and waiting before the power of the Divine. At this point the Goddess appears and leads the figures of her psyche into a new order.

While the novel can be called an account of the process of individuation, it seems specific to women and to the present age. For a woman to find her individuality, she must first experience the destruction of patriarchal rule in her psyche. This change, according to Lessing, is shatteringly difficult, but a necessary one for the archetypal feminine to show forth. The meaning of the intense psychological transmutation seems to be to enable the Goddess to be present in the human psyche of an individual.

Jung has said the hope of a successful crossing into the new age is upon those who can endure individually the process of psychic integration. Lessing strips sweet illusion from the reality of what is required of a person to make this *transitus*. While sobering in its difficulty, her vision proclaims that one may survive.

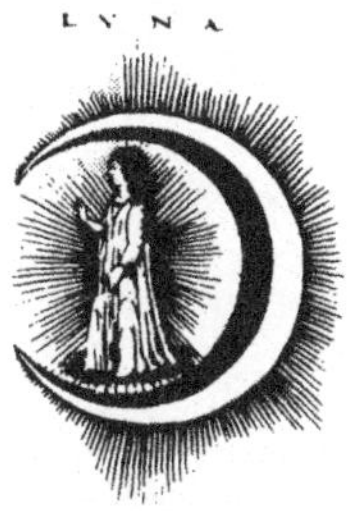

SECTION III

At Bottom—Ereshkigal

At the Bottom

A woman on a path of psychological development walks with the archetypal feminine in ever-widening circles. The feminine is with her from the beginning because she is by virtue of biology and instinct a woman. Her consciousness of the full scope of the archetype is limited, however, by the scant knowledge and awareness of the feminine in the culture. She must look to the ancient past or to the artistic work of women whose lives have traced the steps of the spiral before her, in order to fill in the missing pieces of the character of the archetypal feminine.

The myth of Inanna's descent and Lessing's novel both sketch a similar pattern of a woman's passage from cultural adaptation to an encounter with her essential nature. Both the first section of the descent myth and Lessing's story strip the goddess/woman of all her possessions, all her power, everything which registered in her psyche as a familiar article belonging to her former life. Her dependable habits, her daily chores, her manner of dressing, the objects she cherished, all are gone. She is stripped down to zero.

At this point when she has nothing from before, Ereshkigal appears in person. Ereshkigal operates in the Lessing story as the impersonal, unnameable "it." The stripping takes place in increments in which the characters' lives are more and more ravaged by an impersonal force until nothing is left. At that point, the characters are transformed by an elusive "sweet Presence" who leads the little troop into another order of world. Ereshkigal, in this story, reveals her two sides, the destructive, impersonal "it" and the transforming "sweet Presence."

The Sumerian myth makes more explicit that the goddess who destroys is also the one who transforms. At the point where we left Inanna, she was naked and bowed low. Now she attempts one last act of defiance: she sits on her sister's throne. For her audacity, she is beaten into a piece of rotting meat. Her beaten flesh is hung on a peg where it begins to stink and turn green. A process of transformation has begun, albeit one of putrefaction.

Ereshkigal holds the ultimate power. She must be the goddess of You-Don't-Get-Your-Way. She must be the goddess of death. She must be the goddess of the inevitable turning of the earth on its axis, the inevitable cyclic round of nature grinding on as it has for eons, long before human beings appeared on the planet. Ereshkigal's stripping returns the woman to the bare-bones, essential underpinning of her biological instinctual self.

This return, we discover in the two pieces that follow, quite unexpectedly impels the woman to fall in love with the goddess as Ereshkigal. Lessing hinted at this love story whenever the woman came upon the "sweet Presence" who seemed to hold a promise and who ultimately led her and the others into another world. She does not, however, elaborate on the love of the goddess or describe her gifts. The descent myth hints at Ereshkigal's love for Inanna in that after Inanna's death, the myth tells us Ereshkigal is in the process of giving birth. This synchronistic birth and death implies that Ereshkigal's labor gives birth to the transformed Inanna.

A descent may take place at any spot along the spiral a woman is tracing with her steps. Whenever a descent occurs, it catapults her into the realm of the dark, underworld feminine. She meets there at the bottom a hungry, greedy, ruthless goddess who shakes her to her bones. This goddess demands that she let go of her narrow spectrum of desires, her stunted vision of what life is and can be. The goddess has for her a gift, and it is in the giving and receiving of the gift that the woman falls in love. The gift of the goddess is the full range of the woman's instinctual nature which is the energetic force of her individuality and her creativity. Along with this gift, the goddess infuses the woman with the daring to carry her new vision into the world. The woman in her meeting with the goddess encounters the Self, that is, the archetypal design which carries the essential pattern and meaning of her life. Stripped and laid bare, the woman receives the coherent gift of her true essence. She is essentially, instinctually female, and the goddess infuses her with a fierce, primordial love of femaleness and with the potential for the integration of all her female powers.

The love of femaleness that the meeting with Ereshkigal confers carries the compelling emotion of an archetypal encounter. Being grounded in matter, as any confrontation with Ereshkigal will be, the experience strikes the lower chakras where concrete sexuality resides. A heterosexual woman may be startled to find she is suddenly overwhelmingly attracted to women. A lesbian woman may discover new attitudes of soft acceptance of her body and heightened sexual pleasures. Whichever of the myriad forms the experience may take, the woman is profoundly reborn into a new order of world in which her femaleness occupies the central, focusing position of her emotions and perception.

In her modern version of the descent myth, the play *Queen of Swords,* Judy Grahn (1987) renames Inanna Helen, after the Greek Helen, our ancestress in Western civilization. In the play, Ereshkigal is the proprietress of a lesbian bar. Helen encounters Ereshkigal when she leaves her comfortable middle-class life to explore "undertown." There she meets the gatekeeper of the bar, Nothing, and a chorus of Crow Dike patrons. After passing through the ordeal of the seven gates, her final stripping takes place in a face-to-face meeting with Ereshkigal. In the poetry from the play which follows, Ereshkigal tells Helen who she, Ereshkigal, really is.

The essay on the wounded girl child is the tale of a therapist who, to her surprise, finds herself sexually attracted to women clients. The full scope of the meaning behind these unexpected feelings reveals itself in a dream as an archetypal realignment, an appearance of the goddess on the grave of the dying patriarchs.

No one who has endured a descent will ever treat lightly the suffering it demands. Any descent I know or have heard of is disorienting, emotionally battering, depressing, full of anguish, shame, envy, and despair. A woman may become mad in its wake. Her loss is grievous. Her song is lamentation. May the telling of this myth of Inanna's descent be a map for the initiate, a light of hope to those in the grip of despair, and an orienting matrix to the climbers now ascending from the underworld's dark torment. May the love of Ereshkigal leave on your lips the last line of the myth, "Holy Ereshkigal, sweet is your praise!"

The Descent of Inanna to the Underworld

The Meeting with Ereshkigal

with Inanna bowed low
someone
brings
her
in

her sister stands up
from her wooden throne

Inanna sits on the throne
in her sister's place

the seven Annunaki
judges down below
fix on her the death eye
shout at her the wrath words
cry out SACRILEGE

they beat the doomed woman
into a piece of meat
hang her rotting flesh
on a peg

"Descent to the Butch of the Realm"

by Judy Grahn

Helen

Well, that's all very nice for you.
But what do Lesbians do that has anything
to do with me?

Ereshkigal

Look, Helen! Look into your mind!
If yours is scrambled, look into mine!
You were a goddess before Demeter's time,
Lady Venus of aboveworld form,
Inanna by name, Sumerian born–
you passed through seven gates of the underland
to deliver yourself into my hands,
into Ereshkigal's hands . . .

Helen

And you–who are you, really?

Ereshkigal

I am your wild cherry sister, red and
black sheep sister of the unkempt realm.
I am the Butch of Darkness and the Lady
of the Great Below.
I have a nickname: see if you can guess it.
Thistles in my fur are twisted

---

taut as wily wires of gristle.
You won't find me sitting home in front of TV
drinking beer, not me–I'm outdoors
prowling midnight. Nor do I march
to take back the night with other women
for I never lost it. My name is Shadow of the Wolf,
I woof and I whistle.
My usual companion-lover's name is "Destiny."
She had it tattooed
on my upper arm. She is, of course,
a Dike. She chews me down to something honest
on a weekly basis when I let her.
Oh! But I have plenty of time for you
and your bright beauty–
yes, I have plenty of room for a Venus-type
such as yourself
in my chamber.
Remember me now whenever
you hear the phrase "wild cherry."

Oh descend
Descend to me
to my exhilarating gaze
and my desiring
Yes it is true–I am who wants you
and I hear you have chosen
to come down to me.

Strange to everyone but me that
you would leave the great green rangy
heaven of the american dream,
your husband and your beloved children,
the convenient machines,
the lucky lawn and the possible
picture window–to come down here below.
You left your ladyhood, your queenship, risking
everything, even a custody suit,
even your sanity, even your life. It is
This that tells me you have a warrior

living inside you. It is for this
I could adore you.

Now I want you to enter my stormy regions.
My gatekeeper will guide you; where
do you think you
want to go? Just ask his howling
hollow center.
His name is "Nothingness."
I want you to stand as I stand before you,
tremulous with expectation
as I reach to tangle all my fingers in your hair
to rip away the veil of your
perpetual smile, and then to strip
off your scarf of limitations, even
the birthright of your long hair itself.
Do my stark eyes surprise?
My name is "Naked of Expectations."

And I want to bend you
as I am bent to nip your neck, unclasping
your lapis blue necklace. Ever notice how it
keeps you from talking? You are going to do
a lot of talking. And no small amount of yowling.
Are you certain you should have come?
I may never release you.

Oh descend
Oh lower yourself to love
in the underground, the union
of a woman to one other
woman, not self to self
but self to other
self.

Slap your feet flat on the earth now,
heel first preferably, thrust
your pelvis forward.
You see I am about to change
your center of gravity.

As for those explanatory notes and diagrams
tucked under your arm–put them down.
You won't need them.
You will be too busy with your own internal
computations, as I lick between
your fingers, slipping off the golden rings
of definition and adherence.

Oh descend to me
Lower yourself into yourself
as I go down
and go down
and go down to you.

I want you to fall, as I fall
heavy lying next to you, your twin egg stones
happy underneath my hands, the
pearl-pearl buttons I'm unsnapping,
then that thick-ribbed brassiere that gives you
all the cleavage you have used to
get your men to hope and grope
bearing gifts and favors.
You are your own gift now,
and you have chosen to come to me.

I of the snarled hair, the one earring
and the brassy metallic nailpolish,
I am your wild cherry sister. I am savage,
living in regions ruled by laws
that to you just happen.
When you say "just happen"
you will remember me.

I want you to crawl
unravelling
as I crawl over your dancing belly
to unbuckle the belt of willingness,
last obstacle before you splay your doorway
to my doorway. Reveal to me.
You have a secret self, don't you?

Can you bear your heart to be split
open and to lie so naked
in the sight of
either one of us?

Oh descend to me
mound on mound of Venus meeting
maddened Earth to be unbound on.
Fix your gaze upon me
while I find and flay you
with my fingers and my tongue.

My tongue is nicknamed
"Say Everything."
She's appealing enough
at first until she nails you fast
to solid dirt of the fat earth
and ends your fantasy.

You will moan, Inanna
you will cry.
Everyone you ever were
will die,
while you go down
and go down
and go down
on me.

Hanging helpless on a peg of feeling
as I bear you to your
new and awe-ful place of being, locked in
dead heat, we will argue. We will
fight. Your heart will ooze like red meat.
I will suffer too, to birth you,
to transform and finally release you.
I am cruel, yes. Exacting and not
possibly fooled.
Pain opener. You want pity for your
little yellow egg of being
broken on my greasy griddle.

AT BOTTOM–ERESHKIGAL

I am pitiless. And stirring
I will sear you, so when
next you say "you puking, putrid
lying self-conceited wretch you"
it is my face you will see,
my name you screech out "Oh! I'll Kill!
That Rotten! Bitch!"

Yes, I am the Butch of the Realm, the Lady
of the Great Below. It is hard for me
to let you go.
When next you say "you bitch"–"wild cherry"–
and "it just happens"–
you will think of me
as she who bore you to your new and lawful
place of rising,
took the time and effort
just to get you there
so you could moan Inanna
you could cry
and everyone you ever were
could die.

(A pause. Ereshkigal and Helen embrace, then are surrounded by the Crow Dikes, who hum a love song to them. All collapse to floor.)

Between Woman Analyst and the Wounded Girl Child

For a woman to grow into her fullness, she must find her way to the feminine aspects of the Self. Her ego will then reflect, express, and root in the divine feminine. That is to say, aspects of that complex energy we call the archetypal feminine will inform her ego orientation.

A woman who carries an ill-formed ego due to difficulties in early childhood has particular problems relating to the archetypal feminine. The wound the child sustains from inadequate parenting lives into her adulthood in the form of low self-esteem and an unstable relationship to womanliness and to herself as a woman. This woman's self-worth is further undermined by real and perceived imbalances in the culture in favor of men and the masculine. To the extent that the wounded girl child adapts herself to the culturally more-favored male attitudes and values in order to enhance her self-esteem, she blinds her ego to her natural feminine ground. This woman enters adulthood with a weak ego, dominated by collectively held attitudes to which she clings for survival. Within her psyche she carries a wounded child thwarted in her natural development. Nevertheless, this child carries the seeds of female instinctuality that can lead the woman to the Self.

Much has been written concerning the treatment of the wounded child within the adult in a therapy setting. In this paper I look at one aspect of the transference/countertransference between woman client and woman analyst as that wounded child appears in the analysis and begins to push for integration.

On a larger scale, I am looking at a passage or a crossing over, as a woman shifts the support of her female self from the patriarchy to the archetypal feminine. In this process she will let go of attitudes she has imposed on herself from the outer culture and foster those attitudes spawned by instinct, as these attitudes begin to appear in dreams, imagination, and feeling.

From *Transference/Countertransference*, Nathan Schwartz-Salant and Murray Stein, editors.

On an archetypal scale, this crossing is the task of the shifting age as we move from Pisces to Aquarius. The goddess in her many forms is reemerging into a conscious place in the pantheon. This enormous archetypal event is manifesting itself in myriad ways in our world, not the least of which is its appearance in the unsuspecting, unprepared psyches of analyst and analysand.

Ironically, the very woundedness of the girl child within carries a knowledge of the divine feminine. The wound, while it is seriously incapacitating and emotionally painful to the woman who harbors it, implies a secret loyalty to female instinctuality. The child says through the wound that it is not right for femaleness to be constrained and despised. The restriction of female instinct, self-imposed or culturally imposed, inflames the childhood injury and provides the irritating pressure which may spur the woman toward her own healing.

Woman's secret, sometimes her shame, is that she is linked by blood to the banished Whore of Babylon as well as to Mary the Mother of God. The woman intimately feels instinctual aspects of the feminine that have been repressed and denied by the culture. The archetypal patriarchal backdrop to our culture manifests itself with a stubborn conservatism. As the new archetypal mode–the goddess–emerges, it necessarily appears first in the psyches of individuals who must suffer the weight of it within an alien or hostile culture. The old cultural forms, like a bad marriage or a neurotic defense, tend to live on past their usefulness.

The particular problem for women who are trying to foster and nourish a wounded girl child is that this child ultimately must be grounded in the feminine instinctual aspects of the Self. Feminine instinctuality in the culture often lives in unsavory places. The witch has carried it with her intuitive wisdom and psychic healing. Outrageous women have carried it as they fling their proud sexuality in the face of the proper fathers. Certain collective manifestations of the feminine have been split off and ostracized from viable cultural expression just as they are split off in individual psyches. Little wonder, then, that women tremble when the goddess appears with her promise to heal the wounded child because she enlivens female instinct and demands that it be lived in the world.

I want to look at the blossoming of the seeds of love of the feminine that the wounded child carries. I want to explore a particular transference/countertransference manifestation and some of its implications. I would like to present this situation in the form of a fairy tale. The tale is told from the analyst's point of view, but it could as easily be told from the point of view of any woman.

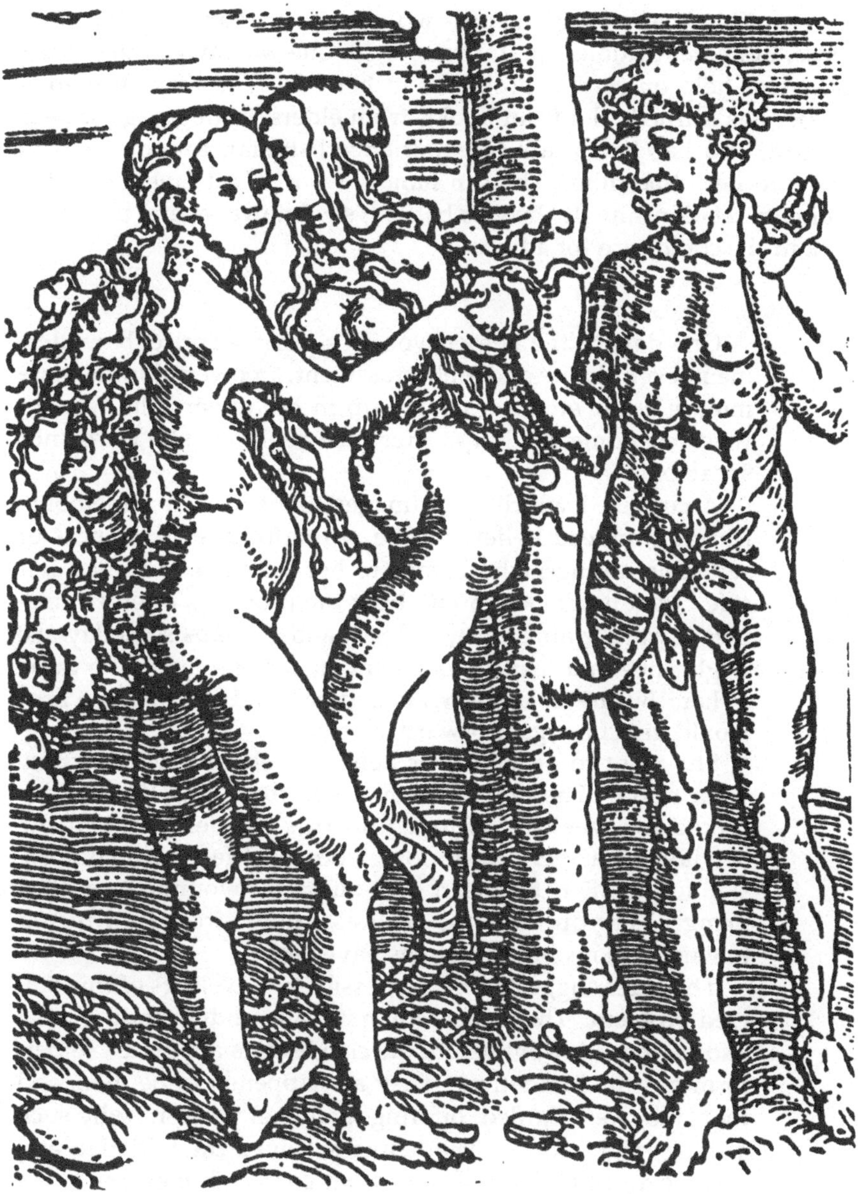

Figure 2. Eve and Lilith with serpent's tail from a woodcut by Lucas Cranach, ca. 1522 (Koltuv 1986, p. 62).

This is a fairy tale about two women working together in a close, intimate relationship. It begins with one woman coming to the other for help on certain problems in her life. The woman who is helper has learned a lot from books, from elders, from going for help herself, and has had years of experience listening to women who come to her. She thinks she can handle what might emerge in this intimate relationship. If she gets baffled, she knows several people to whom she could turn for advice.

One day, to the helper woman's great surprise, bewilderment, even shame and embarrassment, a powerful immediate intense erotic emotion welled up in her toward the woman who has come for help. Her face reddens; she dares not speak of it.

A confused whirling of images follows. She remembers learning, indeed believing, the wrongful destructiveness of seducing anyone who comes to her for help. She had felt safe. Men had talked a lot about the problems of erotic feelings toward women they helped, and perhaps someday she might love in a lustful way some handsome man who came to her. But never in her wildest dream did she imagine Eros would direct her gaze toward a woman.

She went to an elder for help. Surely she would know what to do. The two of them talked for a long time. They talked for weeks. "How could this happen?" asked the bewildered helper. "I do love women. I feel such compassion for women. My heart goes out to the woundedness they bring. Yet you know as well as I how strongly directed toward men my erotic feelings have been."

The elder suggested many possible unravelings of this tangled problem. The helper, still not really understanding what had happened, went before the clan leaders appointed to perform her final initiation. They all happened to be men, and they, too, were baffled, offering many new reasons why such a thing might occur. The helper survived the initiation and became a full-fledged, if somewhat confused, member of the tribe.

The helper settled into her new role. She had a wonderfully rich relationship with the man in her life. Perhaps the feelings she had had toward this woman were "a stage in her development" as the elders had taught her to say. Perhaps she was now in a new phase of her growth, and though she still did not understand what had happened, perhaps the memories of it would fade away.

They did not. Even worse. New women came to her for help. More and more often the burst of erotic feelings arose as these women told their stories. No longer could she console herself that the first experience was a one-time, atypical but necessary, event having to do with a stage in her development. Now her eroticism poured indiscriminately. She never knew toward whom it might flow. She felt in utter despair. "Oh God," she prayed, "must I leave the man I love? What does this mean? Would you have me torn in two?"

As if in answer to her prayer, a great goddess came to her in a dream. She spoke with clarity. "The patriarchy is finished," she said. "Can you not see that? Do you not see the death of it in the two graves you and the other women are preparing? Do you not see the great reed pillar I have implanted on the graves? The reed pillar is my image, my epiphany. Wherever it stands, I am there in all my power. It is my power which stands on the grave of the patriarchy. You must hasten to gather more reeds. Go with the other women. Build the pillars in my image."

The great goddess told her many other things in the dream. "I come to you," she said, "in a very strong form, the erotic. You have forgotten how to love me. I will come to you again and again until you learn. I am teaching you to love me, to love womanliness, to love woman, to love your womanly self. I use strong medicine."

The woman awoke in awe. She felt relieved, felt the revelation was an opening, a beginning, an entrance into a mystery. She began in every way she knew how to worship the great goddess. Slowly, the difficult erotic feelings she had had toward women she helped began to subside. Strangely enough, another phenomenon seemed to appear with their fading. Woman after woman of those who came to her told the following story: "I have always been strongly heterosexual, but the strangest thing is happening . . . ," or, "I have been married twenty-five years, happily, and, suddenly, for no reason, these feelings have arisen . . . ," and always the end of the story was one of a great erotic arousal, as consuming and overwhelming as it was surprising that it was directed toward women.

> The helper bowed in her heart in reverence to the great goddess when she heard these stories, and she blessed the day the goddess had come to her in a dream. She felt the great goddess had focused her sight and clarified difficulties she had suffered all her life.

This tale stands on its own as an example of the healing the archetypal feminine Self can bring and also an example of the hazards passion carries when the feminine erupts in the psyche. The goddess comes in many forms to women. While she offers solid instinctual ground for the wounded child, she carries as well the dangerous allure of any archetype, a temptation for the ego to enfold itself in her power.

As a part of my own attempt to relate to this archetype, I have begun to study the goddess Inanna, the most powerful of the Sumerian goddesses and a precursor to Ishtar and Astarte. I was unaware that Sylvia Perera had also been affected by this goddess. The appearance of Perera's book, *Descent to the Goddess* (1981), and the recent publication by Wolkstein and Kramer (1983) of a new translation of poetry about Inanna suggest that Inanna has something to say to us at this moment.

The poetry about Inanna was written down around 2500 B.C., but the composition of the poems and myths and Inanna's stature as a Mesopotamian goddess predates the writing by at least a thousand years. She carries religious expression of the divine feminine prior to the beginning of the patriarchy and the submitting of the goddess to the monotheistic masculine. That is to say, she carries aspects of the feminine that were repressed by the patriarchy but that women continue to encounter in their deepest instinctual selves. These hidden aspects, then, are part of the feminine ground the wounded child seeks in her effort to be fully woman.

In the myth of Inanna's descent to the underworld, which Perera so ably explores, we learn that Inanna goes to the underworld by her own choice. The first line of the text says, "SHE in great heaven set her ear to great earth." Line four says, "MY LADY left heaven, abandoned earth, went down below." The word for ear in Sumerian also means wisdom or mind. For Inanna to set her ear to the earth and to the underworld is for her to attend to it with her wisdom.

Inanna goes to the underworld to meet her older sister, Ereshkigal, who reigns there. Here, then, is a pattern of the feminine. The upper world goddess, Inanna, the highly cultivated, civilized one, seeks the initiation of the deep and dark primal chthonic powers her older sister holds in the underworld. There Inanna endures a divesting of her power, death, decay, and resurrection.

Another group of poems about Inanna are from the sacred marriage ritual, a New Year's rite. In these poems we find not only the young goddess in all the flutter of courtship and first love but also the bold goddess exalting her body as it longs for sexual fulfillment, and the wise and benevolent goddess who pours her bounty from the "diamond starred" storehouse, the "radiant storehouse of fate." Here are my renditions of three poems in which the goddess exalts her body.

Vulva Song

I, the lady
in the house of holy lapis
in sanctuary I pray
I say a holy prayer

I am the Queen of Heaven
let chanters recite this chant
let singers sing this song
let my bridegroom rejoice with me
let wild bull Dumuzi rejoice

let the words fall out of their mouths
let them sing in the time of their youth
let the song rise up in Nippur
a gift for the son divine

I the Lady sing to praise him
let chanters recite this chant
I Inanna sing to praise him
I give him my vulva song

peg my vulva
my star sketched horn of the Dipper
moor my slender boat of heaven
my new moon crescent cunt beauty

I wait an unplowed desert
fallow field for the wild ducks
my high mound longs for the floodlands

my vulva hill is open
this maid asks who will plow it
vulva moist in the floodlands
the queen asks who brings the ox

the king, Lady, will plow it
Dumuzi, king, will plow it

plow then man of my heart
holy water-bathed loins

holy Ninegal[1] am I

Holy Song

this song is holy

let me tell you where I'm coming from
my vulva is
the power place
a royal sign

I rule with cunt power
I see with cunt eyes
this is where
I'm coming from

An[2]
fit me out
with my vulva
I live right here
in this soft slit
I live right here

my field wants hoeing
this is my holy word
a dazzling palace
without its sun
I want you Dumuzi
your bough raised to my cunt
Dumuzi
you belong in this house
I looked at everyone
Dumuzi I call you
it's you I want
for prince

---

[1]Another name for Inanna.
[2]God of heaven.

Dumuzi, beloved of Enlil[3]
even my mother and father adore you

listen
I will scrub my skin with soap
I will rinse all over with water
I will dry myself with linen
I will lay out mighty love clothes
    I know how exactly
I will look so fine
I will make you feel like a king

Poem in Woman's Tongue[4]

the Good City temple
Eridu temple
is fixed up right

the Moon God temple
temple of Sin
shines radiant

An's temple
Eanna
is armed to protect the day

cloudlike Ezida
head of temples
overflows with blessing for you

GOOD IS THE NAME WE GIVE THIS DAY
DAY OF THE LAPIS BED

holy fire god
holy Gibil
purifies the great sacred room
sanctifies it fit for a queen
fills the reed house
cleans the storehouse
pours the sacred water blessing

he wakes the sleeping day
by shouting its name

---

[3]God of air.
[4]This poem was written in eme-sal, a dialect of Sumerian used for the speech of goddesses and their servants.

AT BOTTOM–ERESHKIGAL

LOOK
THE DAY OF THE BED

the Day the lord exalts the woman
the Day she gives life to her lord
she gives harvest power to her lord
gives the harvest scepter to her lord

SHE WANTS IT
she wants the bed
she wants it

the joy of her heart bed
she wants the bed
she wants it

the sweet thigh bed
she wants the bed
she wants it

the king's bed
she wants the bed
she wants it

the queen's bed
she wants the bed
she wants it

with his sweet thing
with his sweet thing bed
with his sweet thing
the joy of her heart bed
with his sweet thing bed
with his sweet thing

the sweet thigh bed
with his sweet thing bed
with his sweet thing

the king's bed
with his sweet thing bed
with his sweet thing

the queen's bed
with his sweet thing bed
with his sweet thing

she makes the bed for him
she lays out the bed

she makes the bed for him
she lays out the bed

These poems are about one aspect of the goddess, praise of her vibrant body and that of her lover. After the consummation of the marriage, Inanna becomes the gift giver, the weaver of fate, watching over the "house of life." The final words of one of these poems, in which Inanna pours bounty from the storehouse, are "it is strong! it is strong!" Her bounteous gifts nourish, enliven, and strengthen. She is the epitome of fully realized womanhood, strong in itself.

As a way of understanding more deeply the complexity of this goddess, a group of us worked with the poems over a period of months, finally developing a performance piece, which we have presented a few times. The work with the poems has meant many things to us, not the least of which was the delight, the good fun, of women enjoying ribaldry. The underlying experience of the performance, however, was an encounter with the sacred. We put on the robes and roles of priestesses to the goddess and moved through the poems in that basic attitude.

A whole variety of reactions have surfaced from those of us who took part in the performance as well as from people in the audiences who viewed it. The one reaction that comes repeatedly and that pertains to this paper is the conflict between the old gods and the new. Dreams have come that say, on the one hand, that Jehovah unequivocally disapproves of Inanna and what she evokes in women. Other women have dreamed, following our performance, of great violence being done to them by men. All of us have struggled with a sense of shame that we dared to sing exaltation to our bodies in a public place.

On the other hand, powerful eruptions of change have appeared in dreams connected with the performance of the Inanna poems. More than once, these dreams contained an image of a nuclear blast along with images of the woman dreamer leaving behind her former relationship to the collective fathers. I take these dreams to be introducing an image of the new age, the fission which releases a new kind of energy altogether.

For women to leave behind their former daughterly relationship to the patriarchy and ground themselves in their own feminine nature is a shift in loyalty of huge proportion. It reverberates on the personal level, as this woman writes: "It connects me with a small piece of earth on which to plant my soul," while in the past "this flame would leap out briefly, tempt fate, and disappear quickly in shame and fear."

The shift also reverberates archetypally. The reemergence of the goddess, the archetypal feminine, shakes the archetypal status quo. A new face of God appears, and She is a woman. Not without great upheaval will She take her place beside the gods who have enjoyed dominance for 3,000 years.

For certain women, in addition to a cognitive awareness of her appearance, the goddess archetype is an active force in the psyche, coming to them in dreams, fantasies, visions, and feelings. This energy is life changing. It will lead women to carve out new forms for their lives, new channels of expression out in the world of the twentieth and twenty-first centuries. From the energy of the goddess informing their lives, women will discover forms which have no precedents, and these individually carved forms will be the expression of each woman's individual perception. This carving of new forms requires great courage and a devotion to one's individual vision. It requires that one's feet be planted solidly on feminine ground. The visions of individuals will doubtless begin to cluster around common themes, and women will gather in groups and together invent ways to channel their new creative work into the world.

Jung has, in his own life, in his writings, and in his work with patients, exposed the enormous power of archetypal energies in forming and shaping the direction of individual lives and of collective movements. When a great shift is occurring in the archetypal drama, as it is now, the shift, as Jung described it in his book, *Aion* (1951), necessarily produces conflict, not only between people with differing loyalties but also between the voices carried inside oneself. It cannot be otherwise. Perhaps for generations this conflict will continue to manifest itself. I believe we now have the opportunity and the obligation of carrying the conflict with more consciousness of its relationship to the new age, that is, to the struggle of the goddess to achieve Her place in the godhead.

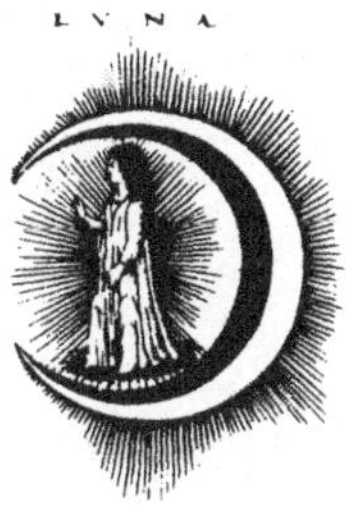

SECTION IV
Ascent from Below

The Eye of Death

Our goddess, Inanna, has met Ereshkigal and hangs rotting on a peg within Ereshkigal's sight. Only now do we learn that Ereshkigal is pregnant and lies moaning, presumably in labor. One goddess dies, and another is giving birth. The god/woman hangs on a wooden stake, and her tormentor is the source of new life and resurrection.

The parallels to the Christian myth are astounding. However, in this version the two gods, Inanna and Ereshkigal, are female, and the crucified god, Inanna, comes out of the underworld with a new way of seeing. She has picked up some of Ereshkigal's charm. Accompanying her is a demonic clear-sightedness, an impersonal cutting through ego centeredness, sentimentality, and nostalgia. Most important of all, she now carries the very eye of death. Inanna is transformed into a goddess who can move back and forth between her former highly civilized self and her new fierce, demanding, precise vision of the primacy of raw nature. Her heart has been seared in the purifying fire of primordial reality. She carries Ereshkigal in her bones.

The essay on the Thesmophoria that follows describes a ritual enactment of the descent theme from another part of the world, Greece and Old Europe. In this ritual, all of the women are menstruating. Menstrual bleeding becomes the center point, the focus, a metaphorical lesson in the meaning of descent.

What a bloody mess! All these menstruating women shouting, wielding knives, carving up piglets, digging their hands into rotten, putrid pig's flesh, laughing hilariously as they eat little crescent cookies the shape of the huge pudenda on their altar. They are all bleeding, and on the solemn day of fasting they bleed together into the fields. Every year they came, for centuries, to reenact, to glorify descent.

The women, by enacting the Thesmophoria, were holding a psychological content, a wisdom, an acknowledgment essential to the on-goingness of life as they knew it. Menstrual bleeding was primary. Were they not then stripped of the encrustations of persona, of hierarchy, of position? Each was primarily and simply her organs of sex and reproduction. Bloody buildup and flow, buildup and flow. Each woman was reduced to the common autonomous cyclic process of the physical workings of her body. In the ritual, she gave over everything to this sovereign process that keeps all life going at its basic physical level. In the Thesmophoria, this sovereign is known as Snake. In the descent myth, she is Ereshkigal.

The ritual was a teaching essential to the life of women and essential to the life of the community. Each year the women gathered into their hands the rot indispensable to the cycles of life, planted it with seeds in the fields which already held their sloughed-off blood. By enduring the ritual, they confirmed for another year their ability to descend into the chaos of disintegrating decay and emerge with the nourishing product of transformation. They affirmed their ability to hold in consciousness both primary nature and cultural achievement. That is, they acknowledged their utter dependence on the physical workings of nature with its constant threat of disaster, side by side with their hard won community achievements, their development of culture, their tending and care of families and government and art and production.

Both rituals, Inanna's descent and the Thesmophoria, bring up from the dark of the underworld the primacy of matter. Without matter, spirit would not exist. To live in the world of spirit and ignore matter is a hubris that begs a downfall. The world of human achievement, including the achievements of individual development, is forever in danger of being grabbed from behind by the overpowering force of the unconscious, by a turn of fate, by limitation, by illness, death, natural disasters. These ancient women guarded consciousness of matter's hold on them by the enactment of ritual.

The descent myth has its uprising also. Inanna is brought back to life. Ninshubur, who has watched over Inanna's descent, persuades the earth god of sweet waters, Enki, to rescue the goddess.

His messengers, the galaturra and the kurgarra, trick Ereshkigal into giving them her body. They sprinkle over her the water of life and the plant of life, and Inanna is revived.

After agreeing to send someone down in her place, Inanna leaves the underworld. But the transformed Inanna has little demons clinging to her side. These creatures carry Inanna's new consciousness. They are child snatchers, bride killers, inhuman, amoral rascals, like Ereshkigal herself. Inanna has incorporated Ereshkigal's eye of death as a new comprehension of the primacy of nature. She sees clearly that human beings are at the mercy of forces inconceivably larger than they, forces which operate entirely without human caring. She has taken Ereshkigal into herself. Now she is both a caring goddess, witness how she cares for Ninshubur, and a goddess who has the capacity to stare with the eye of death. Her first victim is her husband, Dumuzi. In his hubris, he has not mourned Inanna. Clearly he does not yet understand the full force and autonomy of Ereshkigal's realm. He must descend to the underworld to gain this consciousness.

The persistence of this mythic theme over thousands of years attests to its place in the bedrock of the archetypal structure of the psyche. Its complexities and nuances, its many layers light up the imagination. Each one who reads it brings a new story to mold into its basic design. The descent stands as an invitation to measure the steps you have taken down your own path, and as a whole pattern that repeats in women's lives with ever-deepening, ever-widening consequence.

The Descent of Inanna to the Underworld

The Ascent

IV

three days and three nights pass
Ninshubur
Chosen Mistress
remembers
her Lady's word

wails for her
cries in lamentation by the ruins
plays a drum song
drums for her in the throne court
wanders for her
wanders through the houses of the gods

tears at her eyes
tears at her mouth
tears at the place she shows no one

wears rags for her
only rags

sets her feet towards Enlil's house
goes alone to Enlil's house
Great Mountain Temple
Ekur
enters Great Mountain Ekur house
looks him in the eye and
WEEPS

says
    father Enlil
    do not let anyone
    hold your daughter down below

do not let your
good silver
mix with the dust of that place

do not let your
precious lapis lazuli
be split with the mason's stone

do not let your
sweet boxwood
be sawn with the carpenter's wood

do not let the maiden
Inanna
be held down below

Enlil enraged
says to Ninshubur

my daughter wants great heaven
wants great earth below

Inanna wants great heaven
wants great earth below

forbidden are those desires
desires for netherworld powers

who seizes them
must stay there
down below

who would ever want to come back
from that place anyway

Enlil does not help her
she goes to Ur

in Ur
Nanna's temple
Moon God temple
House-of-Light
Ekishnugal
goes to Nanna
looks him in the eye and
WEEPS

says
    father Nanna
    do not let anyone
    hold your daughter down below

    do not let your
    good silver
    mix with the dust of that place

    do not let your
    precious lapis lazuli
    be split with the mason's stone

    do not let your
    sweet boxwood
    be sawn with the carpenter's wood

    do not let the maiden
    Inanna
    be held down below

Nanna enraged
says to Ninshubur

    my daughter wants great heaven
    wants great earth below

    Inanna wants great heaven
    wants great earth below

forbidden are those desires
desires for netherworld powers

who seizes them
must stay there
down below

who would ever want to come back
from that place anyway

Nanna does not help her
she goes to Eridu

in Eridu
enters the temple of Enki
looks him in the eye and
WEEPS

says
father Enki
do not let anyone
hold your daughter down below

do not let your
good silver
mix with the dust of that place

do not let your
precious lapis lazuli
be split with the mason's stone

do not let your
sweet boxwood
be sawn with the carpenter's wood

do not let the maiden
Inanna
be held down below

Enki says
to Ninshubur

my daughter
what has she done
I am deeply troubled

Inanna
what has she done
I am deeply troubled

mistress of all the lands
what has she done
I am deeply troubled

sacred woman of An
what has she done
I am deeply troubled

he takes dirt
from under his fingernail
makes a *kurgarra*

he takes dirt
from a second fingernail
makes a *galaturra*

he gives to the *kurgarra*
the life-giving plant

he gives to the *galaturra*
the life-giving water

Enki says
to the *galaturra*
to the *kurgarra*

GO
creep into the netherworld

at the great wooden door
fly around like flies
sneak through the door cracks like demons

there Ereshkigal
great with child
lies moaning

no linen covers
her pure body

nothing binds
her full-vessel breasts

she rakes at her body
with ax-sharp claws

her hair tangles on her head
like leeks

when she cries
　　my womb-heart
　　oh my womb-heart

say to her
　　our Lady
　　you are troubled
　　oh your poor womb-heart

when she moans
　　my liver-soul
　　oh my liver-soul

say to her
　　our Lady
　　you are troubled
　　oh your poor liver-soul

then she will say
    WHO ARE YOU
    who cries with the pain in my womb-heart
    who moans with the pain in my liver-soul

    if you are gods
    let me promise you something

    if you are men
    let me change your fate

make her swear to this
by the breath of heaven
by the life of earth

stay then
now you are safe

even if she offers you
a river to drink
do not accept it

even if she offers you
a field of grain to eat
do not accept it

say to her
    give us the beaten flesh
    hanging on that peg

she will answer
    that beaten flesh
    is your *queen*!

say
    whether our king
    or our queen
    give it to us

she will give you
the beaten flesh
hanging on the peg

spread
over the flesh
the life-giving plant

pour
over the flesh
the life-giving water

Inanna
will
rise up

the *galaturra*
the *kurgarra*
obey Enki's words

at the great wooden door
they fly around like flies
they sneak through the door cracks like demons

Ereshkigal
great with child
lies moaning

no linen covers
her pure body

nothing binds
her full-vessel breasts

she rakes at her body
with ax-sharp claws

her hair tangles on her head
like leeks

when she cries
my womb-heart
oh my womb-heart

they say to her
our Lady
you are troubled
oh your poor womb-heart

when she moans
my liver-soul
oh my liver-soul

they say to her
our Lady
you are troubled
oh your poor liver-soul

she says
WHO ARE YOU
who cries with the pain in my womb-heart
who moans with the pain in my liver-soul

if you are gods
let me promise you something

if you are men
let me change your fate

they make her swear
by the breath of heaven
by the life of earth

they stay there
now they are safe

she offers them
a river to drink
they do not accept it

she offers them
a field of grain to eat
they do not accept it

they say to her
    give us the beaten flesh
    hanging on that peg

pure Ereshkigal
answers
the *galaturra*
the *kurgarra*
    that beaten flesh
    is your *queen!*

they say
    whether our king
    or our queen
    give it to us

she gives them
the beaten flesh
hanging on the peg

one spreads
over her
the life-giving plant

one pours
over her
the life-giving water

INANNA
RISES UP

holy Ereshkigal
says
to the *galaturra*
to the *kurgarra*
    carry
    your queen
    away

V

Inanna
leaves the netherworld

the plan of Enki
freed her

on her way
as she is leaving
the Annunaki seize her

    stop
they say
    no one can leave
    the netherworld
    unscathed

    Inanna
    for you to leave
    give us
    a head
    for your head

holy Inanna
comes up

a man walks before her
he is not a deputy
but he carries a staff

a man walks behind her
he is not a soldier
but he carries arms

small demons like fence reeds
large demons like fence posts
surround her
cling to her side

the men walking with her
the men with Inanna
know no food
know no drink

eat no offerings of flour
drink no offerings of water
accept no offerings of gifts

are never held in the
sweet legs of a spouse
tear the spouse
from the lap of her husband

never kiss a sweet child
snatch the child from the nurse
the bride from her wedding bed

Inanna
returns from the netherworld

Ninshubur
drops
at her feet

wears rags
rolls in the dust

the demons
shout at pure Inanna
    go
    Inanna
    to your city

    we will
    take
    this one
    away

pure Inanna
answers
 this is my faithful mistress
 my good-word bearer
 carrier of true words

 she obeyed what I said
 did not forsake
 the word I spoke

 she wailed for me
 cried in lamentation by the ruins
 played a drum song
 drummed for me in the throne court
 wandered for me
 wandered through the houses of the gods

 tore at her eyes
 tore at her mouth
 tore at the place she shows no one

 wore rags for me
 only rags

 set her feet towards Enlil's house
 went alone to Ekur

 she went alone
 to Nanna
 Moon Temple in Ur

 she went alone
 to Eridu
 entered the temple of Enki

she is the one
who gave me
my life
I will
never
give her
to you

let's go
let's go to Umma
to the temple Sigkursaga
brickworks-inside-the-mountain

at Sigkursaga
in Umma
Shara
drops
at her feet

wears rags
rolls in the dust

the demons
shout
at pure Inanna

go
Inanna
to your city

we will
take
this one
away

pure Inanna
answers
    Shara
    sings my praises
    Shara
    cuts my nails
    combs my hair

    I will
    never
    give him
    to you

let's go
let's go to Badtibira
to the temple Emushkalamma
land's halo temple

at Emushkalamma
in Badtibira
Lulal
honey-man
drops at her feet

wears rags
rolls in the dust

the demons
shout
at pure Inanna

    go
    Inanna
    to your city

    we will
    take
    this one
    away

pure Inanna
answers
    Lulal
    who stands at my right
    Lulal
    who stands at my left

    I will
    never
    give him
    to you

let's go
let's go to Kullab in the steppe
let's go
to the great apple tree

they follow her
to Kullab
to the great apple tree
in the steppe

there Dumuzi
her husband
sits on a splendid throne
wears a magnificent robe

the demons
grab at his thighs
seven
pour milk from his churn
demons lunge at him
smite his head

he is stricken
the shepherd
lays down
his long reed flute
Dumuzi
lays down
his single-reed pipe

Inanna
stares
the death eye

speaks
the wrath words

cries out
SACRILEGE

says
CARRY
HIM
AWAY

gives
Dumuzi
into their hands

the men who walk with him
the men with Dumuzi
know no food
know no drink

eat no offerings of flour
drink no offerings of water
accept no offerings of gifts

are never held in the
sweet legs of a spouse
tear the spouse
from the lap of her husband

never kiss a sweet child
snatch the child from the nurse
the bride from her wedding bed

Dumuzi cries out
turns pale

raises his hands to heaven
to Utu

O Utu
you are my wife's brother
I am your sister's husband

I am spouse
of a goddess
I am not mortal

I carried
oil
to your mother's house

I carried
milk
to Ningal's house

I have danced
on Inanna's knee

make my hand
the hand of a snake

make my foot
the foot of a snake

help me
escape these demons
don't let them hold me

Utu
hears
his cry

he makes his hand
the hand of a snake

he makes his foot
the foot of a snake

Dumuzi
escapes
the demons

slithering snake
through fields, over mountains
gets away to Geshtinanna
his sister Geshtinanna

Geshtinanna sees him
tears at her cheeks
tears at her mouth

tends Dumuzi's wounds
wraps him in a cloak
cries in lamentation for her brother

> brother
> O my brother
> no life left before you
>
> brother
> O my brother
> no wife
> no children
>
> brother
> O my brother
> no friend
> no companion
>
> brother
> O my brother
> no comfort for our mother

demons scatter
search for Dumuzi

small demons say
to large demons

demons have no mother
no father no mother
no sister no brother
no wife no child

demons snatch people
cling to their sides

demons know no kindness
know no good from evil
demons ponder
how will a man
all alone
save himself

he will not go to a friend
he will not go to his in-laws
he will go to his sister
to the house of Geshtinanna

the demons
clap their hands
scatter
search for the shepherd

Geshtinanna sings her last cry
demons appear at her door

take us to your brother

Geshtinanna speaks not a word

the demons
spread disease
on her loins

Geshtinanna speaks not a word

the demons
scratch at her face

Geshtinanna speaks not a word

the demons spread disease
on her buttocks

Geshtinanna speaks not a word

the demons
pour tar
on her lap

Geshtinanna speaks not a word

let's go
let's go to the sheepfold
to the pure sheepfold of Dumuzi

demons find him
surround him
torture him
seize him
tear apart his sheepfold

Geshtinanna
wanders in the city
a lost bird
crying for her brother

brother
O my brother
let me
take this sorrow for you

brother
O my brother
let the demons
take me
in your place

Dumuzi
is weeping

the queen
Inanna
finds him

Inanna
take his hand

says
    half the year will be yours
    Dumuzi
    half the year your sister's

    on the day you set
    your sister will be seized

    on the day your sister sets
    that day
    you will be seized

Inanna
gives Dumuzi
in her place

HOLY ERESHKIGAL
SWEET IS YOUR PRAISE

The Thesmophoria

A Women's Ritual

You dream of menstruation. You dream of hemorrhaging, of flooding, of staining your clothes, of spotting. You dream of having your period with your friends, with your mother, with your daughters. You dream of other women flowing, staining, hemorrhaging. You dream of welcoming the flow, of hating it, of being embarrassed, of hiding.

You gather memories of menstruation. You remember seeing blood in the toilet, but you cannot remember what your mother said about it. You remember she called the red sheet stain fingernail polish.

You remember Jean Ann, Grady, Nancy, and Jo Ellen bending over the dictionary on the den floor at Charlotte's house. They are looking up the WORD. You think it starts with an "a," "administration." They laugh. "No! Menstruation!" They are talking about something you have never heard of, something as dirty as fucking.

You are the last one to start your period. You have taped a toilet paper pad on your bride doll. You feel your face, your groin flush when you play this game with her.

Your period starts. You are in the pink bathroom. Your mother is outside hanging sheets on the clothesline. You tell her you think you have started your period. Neither of you has ever spoken that word between you.

She comes inside with you. She does not say much. She says, "Sometimes it is a relief when it starts." You wonder what she is talking about.

You are walking home from school with Jean Ann. She has on her red teddy bear coat. Something drops. "Look over there," she says. She picks the something up. You do not see what it is because you were looking where she pointed. Later she tells you her Kotex fell off.

Reprinted with permission from *Psychological Perspectives,* vol. 17, no. 1 © 1986 by the C. G. Jung Institute of Los Angeles (10349 W. Pico Blvd., Los Angeles, CA 90064).

You menstruate for thirty-four years. After you have stopped menstruating, you hear your friends talking about having their periods. You realize you are now set apart from them. You dream that you need to make a ritual marking the passage from having periods to their ceasing. You cannot think what to do.

You begin to see yourself as a nonmenstruating woman. Walking down the street, you notice the women who still menstruate. In cafes you watch them. You sense the cycle going on in their bodies. You sense the trembling edge of their fertility. Your body begins to tingle. You feel tears pressing behind your eyes. You feel a surge of caring for them. You have an urge to protect them in their vulnerability.

You hear that Northwest Indian women menstruate sitting on the ground on soft moss. Carol says she was at a cabin alone once and wanted to menstruate into the earth. She could not bring herself to do it. You hear of a woman who owns a beaded African gourd used to collect menstrual blood. Judy says she would like to collect her menstrual blood, but she does not know what she would do with it. Nyla says the blood is good for plants. She knows a woman who puts menstrual blood on her plants, and the plants flourish.

You hear that in the past women's ritual centered around the mystery of the blood. You learn that women celebrated the connection between the fertility cycle in their bodies and the fertility cycle of the earth. You learn that the women honored their menstrual cycle as a gift from the deity. You learn that women fiercely protected the sacredness of their fertility. You feel the power of a ritual gathering of women, articulating and celebrating the mystery we carry in our bodies. You want to know more about the sacred ritual we have lost.

The fields belong to woman. In her body, woman carries the secret knowledge of fertility and growing. Woman is like the field. The field and the woman both caress the seed. The seed is at home in her body and in the earth's body. The seed feeds off the moist nurturing food her blood carries and the earth carries. Her body naturally harbors the seed in her womb. The seed grows. The mystery astounds her. And she is the mystery. Wisely, the fields belong to woman.

Long before the Olympians came to power, led by the great patriarch, Zeus, the women in Greece celebrated the Thesmophoria. Each year at the time of planting, the women gathered to remember the sacred mystery of the seed in the earth and the seed in their bodies. No one knows the ritual's beginning. Votive remains, similar to those used in the Thesmophoria, have been found in all parts of Old Europe dating from 6000 B.C. (Burkert 1985, p. 13; Gimbutas 1982, pp. 214, 215).

The ritual is of "immemorial antiquity" (Harrison 1962, p. 120). From the time women discovered that wild seeds gathered could be saved, could be buried in the earth, could grow, they began to bless the seeds with blood and flesh. They celebrate the ritual which in Greece became the Thesmophoria.

Women who take part in the Thesmophoria have reached the age of the beginning of their menstrual cycle. They have blossomed, have borne or can bear children. They share the common bond in their bodies of the ripe pear of a womb filling and shedding blood with the moon. Or they have passed beyond the menses. They have survived childbirth, disease, miscarriage, hardship, famine, sorrow, turmoil. They have passed the climacteric, and the memory of the bleeding, the blood memory, mixes with time to form wisdom.

For the young girls who do not yet menstruate, the Greeks hold a separate rite called the Arretophoria. Girls between the ages of seven and eleven participate. In the Arretophoria the girls enact parts of the ritual drama of the Thesmophoria, but the mystery is carefully hidden. Four girls of noble birth lodge during the festival in the temple of the goddess. On one of the nights, the girls carry sacred objects which cannot be named and cannot be seen. Women place the objects in baskets which the four girls carry on their heads. They walk down a natural underground passage. At the bottom of the descent, they exchange the sacred objects for something else that is wrapped and hidden. This they bring back to the temple. Thus the young girls begin their preparation for the central mystery of their lives which they will later celebrate in the festival of the Thesmophoria (Harrison 1962, pp. 131-133).

The ritual of the Thesmophoria begins with three days of preparation, during which the women observe rites of purification. For three preparatory days and nights, the women abstain from sexual intercourse (Burkert 1985, p. 244). Thus they begin their withdrawal from men. In their houses, the women sleep alone; they prepare cots on which to sleep away from the marriage bed. The women begin to work and walk alone. They begin to enter wholly into the femaleness of themselves. They eat garlic to repel the men by the unappetizing smell of their breath. They carefully place a garlic supper for Hecate on her piles of stones at crossroads.

At dusk on each of the three preparatory days, the women gather at the chosen fields (Burkert 1985, p. 242). There they build the huts in which they will sleep during the nights of the ritual. There they prepare the great altar. Each woman constructs her own hut (Burkert 1985, p. 107). She brings from the countryside great branches of the wild fig, the tree which in Greece designates the entrance to the underworld (Harrison 1962, p. 136). She covers her shelter with branches of the wild fig. Inside her hut, she prepares a couch for herself of grasses and soft piles of leaves.

Over the hut and on the couch she strews the lygos plant. She weaves its twigs around the hut's opening. She secures its leaves and flowers into the walls over her couch. In a ceremony after the work is finished each evening, the women gather near the alter and sip a cooling drink of crushed lygos leaves.

The women tell many stories about the lygos plant. They say lygos flowers in three colors by the river Imbrasos, or Parthenios. They say lygos grows on the island of Samos, or Parthenia, Island of the Virgin. They say lygos grows profusely on the sandy flats of the river bank, its blue, white, and pale red flowers appearing in countless numbers. Here among the lygos Hera would come to pass her katamenia, her menstrual period. Here the women of Samos would bring each month the statue of Hera from her temple and pass the katamenia with her. Afterwards, the women would bathe Hera and return with her to the temple, virginal (Kerényi 1975, pp. 154-159).

In preparation for the Thesmophoria, the women drink the lygos drink to urge on the menses. The leaves of the lygos plant tremble on the branches at the doors of the huts, a sign of the impending flow. The droplets of blood begin to loosen in the walls of the women's wombs, begin to gather in silent streams. From the first show of the blood, the women are sanctified for the great Thesmophoria. They tie a red band around their arms, telling the others they are ready, flowing, set apart, untouchable because sacred. The flow of this month of sowing, Pyanepsion, is holy, belonging to the deities who rule the Thesmophoria (Burkert 1985, p. 245).

The day of the festival arrives. The women gather at the sacred field. Only the women gather. Not even a male dog is allowed. The women guard the area with sacrificing knives, roasting-spits, and torches. Once, women with blood-smeared faces castrated a man caught spying (Burkert 1985, p. 244).

The first day of the three-day festival is called both Kathodos and Anodos, downgoing and uprising. The women, purified in the three days of preparation, carry down into a chasm newborn suckling

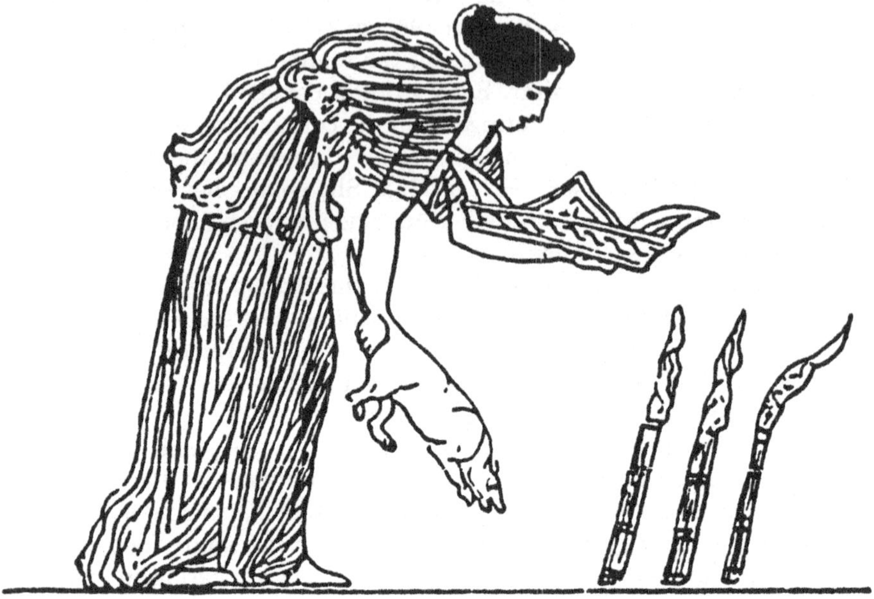

Figure 3. A vase painting from a lekthos in the National Museum at Athens, possibly depicting the Thesmophoria.

pigs. Squealing and wiggling, the piglets struggle in the strong arms of the women. Together they descend into the chasm.

The same day, the women climb out of the chasm carrying great heaps of rotted pig's flesh. The sacred nature of this ritual silenced any report of what actually happened down below. That the women killed the pigs is certain. The source of the rotted flesh, which they carry out the same day, is unknown. Some say the flesh remained from the pig slaughter the year before. Some say the rotted flesh belonged to pigs sacrificed during the spring threshing ritual. Some say the transformation of the sweet flesh to rotten meat is a mystery.

The little pigs, they say, were food for the great underground primal deities, the snakes. The snake deity carries life itself under the earth, rules the mystery of the deep earth. The women bring food to the great snake deity, little piglets with their fat and fertile propensity.

The women bow before great Snake in wonder. They are inexorably bound to Snake, even when they do not know it or do not acknowledge it, for Snake is the power in the earth, in the field, and the power in the bodies of the women.

The women honor Snake with sacrifice. Each woman descends into the chasm with a pig for Snake. The pig is a promise to Snake, a promise that yearly seals the bond between Snake and woman. Snake does not need to be reminded of her power, but the women! Ah! They tend to forget. When life is going well in the village and the storehouse is full, the women might say, "How clever we are! How well we provide for our people!" They might forget that the power of life belongs to Snake. To remember this, they celebrate the Thesmophoria.

The women are fond of the little pigs with creamy pink skin soft as a baby's. Each woman brings her pick of the litter, the feistiest, healthiest, roundest little pig, takes it to Snake at the Thesmophoria. At the bottom of the chasm, near the sacred abode of Snake, the women kill the pigs. They slit open the pigs' bellies (Burkert 1985, p. 234, fn. 14). It is hard for the women to do and pains them. The little pigs become part of them. The women say to Snake, "Here! Here is little pig! She is a part of me! She with her ripening cunt, her estrus, her great belly waiting for seeds! Here she is! Now, Snake, I give her to you! She belongs to you anyway. It is you who stir life in our wombs. At this moment I know the life you sustain in my body. Great Snake! Mystery! Eat!"

They say the snakes eat almost all of the pig flesh (Burkert 1985, p. 243).

The women climb out of the chasm carrying baskets of the rotted flesh of pigs. The rattling and hissing sounds a snake makes accompany the women climbing. They carry in baskets the transformed food of Snake. They make the sounds of Snake. The women have become Snake. Snake enlivens the women, incarnates in the women. Snake is alive and emerges into the upper world inside the bodies of the women.

The second day of the Thesmophoria is called Nesteia, the Middle Day, the day of the solemn fast. The only substance eaten is the red-fleshed seed of the pomegranate. Should a seed drop on the ground, it remains there for the dead. Silence and gloom pervade the atmosphere (Burkert 1985, p. 244).

On this middle day, the women mix the rotten pigs' flesh with seed corn. They place the mixture on the great altar. There it remains in the sacred place throughout the day.

In bringing up from the chasm a portion of the rotten flesh, the women have taken food from Snake. As compensation for this removal, they now carry down a substitute. They make sacred images whose names may not be spoken. They form the images from cereal paste and carry them down in baskets into the chasm. The *sacra* whose names may not be spoken look like penises and scrota or like coiled snakes.

The remainder of the day, the women fast seated on the ground. It is said that the women imitate the ancient way of life. They move into the primitive way their grandmothers knew. They sit upon the ground. They sit in ritual silence in the sacred fields (Harrison 1962, p. 127).

Silently their own blood flows into the fields. They sit cunt to earth, kiss the sweet soil of the fields. The blood of the women flows into the field. The soil of the field drinks the rich blood of the women. In solemn silence the women give to the earth their own substance. Snake moves through the women in the blood flow. Snake carries the fertilizing blood richness into the earth's body. The women are one with the earth. The life of the earth and the life of the women comingle, an open exchange, a bond of kin, revitalized by the mysterious power of Snake.

The fast is broken at sunset. In a ritual gathering, the women eat sacred cakes. The cakes are replicas of the great pudenda that sits on the altar (Burkert 1985, p. 244). The silence is broken. The women begin to joke and to laugh as they pass to one another the little cakes in the shape of a cunt, a slender crescent, a half moon.

In the evening, the women gather around the fire. The jovial mood which began after the fast was broken now swells to hilarity. The presence of Snake in the women sweeps away the boundaries of ordinary life. Gone are the daily concerns which bind the women to the life of the village: the care of children, lovers, husbands, gossip, struggle. The women have severed their ties to daily life and begin to see with the pitiless eyes of Snake.

The vision loosens their tongues. They tell what they see. Passion stirs and rises. They begin to shout at each other. What has been tolerated, ignored, hidden, is exposed. They hurl scurrilous remarks, scathing, burning descriptions that imagine details of acts of utmost privacy. No one is spared, not the women, not their parents, relatives, husbands, lovers, friends. They laugh. They jeer. The one who is shouting vies to outdo the last. They rage. They cry. They fight, hurl clods and stones (Burkert 1985, p. 104; Harrison 1962, p. 136).

No one is spared. Secrets, grudges, hatreds, envies, jealousies, all are exposed. A woman cannot avoid seeing her secret self made public, her dark and hidden passions flung in the air by the voices of the shouting women. The shouting exposes secrets, shatters pride, levels the women to a common ground.

The women are mortified. They are stripped of pride, shaken and leveled. The tongue of Snake cuts away foolish pride, foolish desire. They acknowledge all belongs to Snake, and no one of them creates, loves, works, builds, plays outside the life-sustaining embrace of Snake.

One by one they begin to walk towards their huts. Each goes to her own hut to sleep. Each carefully strews lygos over her couch. The lygos which brings on the blood flow is said to be hostile to reptiles (Harrison 1962, p. 130). Each woman knows that the intimate contact with Snake is double-edged. Snake's gifts of sight and fecundity are only a thin line removed from her powers of wild possession and madness. The women protect themselves with the lygos at night when their heightened daytime alertness fades into sleep. They ask Snake to guard them from madness and possession, acknowledging that madness, too, is her power.

The third day of the festival is called Kallegeneia, Fair Born of Fair Birth. The women awake singing. They have survived the great trials of the Thesmophoria.

They have dared to enter the abode of Snake. They have sacrificed before her. They have participated in a ritual death in her presence. Snake has filled them. The deity herself has risen from the depths in the bodies of the women. Her awesome power possessed them. She loosened the boundaries of ordinary life and shook the women.

Now the day of the Fair Born arrives. Snake returns to her chasm. Now the women move about, sensing her withdrawal. The air is clear. The air is no longer shaking. Snake has departed.

The old hierarchy returns. The older women approach the altar, the honored ones who have slept many years on the lygos. The women gather around them. The old ones speak of Snake's departure. We are left with her memory, they say. They lift the baskets of seed-flesh off the altar and pass among the women. Each woman takes a portion of the mixture and follows the basket carriers into the field. There the women bury the seed-flesh in the sanctified soil (Harrison 1962, Chapter IV). When all the seeds are planted, the women stand in the plowed rows. Softly they begin to sing. Whatever name they give to the great snake deity, they sing her praise. From time immemorial they sing to her. She has had many names. Few have survived to us.

In ancient Sumer, she was called Ereshkigal, and the women sang:

> Holy Ereshkigal
> sweet is your praise

Where in modern life can women find a place to praise the great snake deity? She is lost here. There is no place for her. We have not received memory of her from our mothers. We have forgotten how to pass knowledge of her to our daughters. No sacred festival honors the central mystery of our lives. Our mothers are ashamed to speak of it.

Our tradition is gone. The memory is shattered. We gather only broken pieces. We have forgotten which pieces belong together. We have forgotten that the same deity rules the descent to the underworld and the mysterious cycle in our bodies. We have forgotten that descent must have its sacrifice. We have forgotten that the rotten substance of the sacrifice is a gift of fecundity.

In the festival of the Thesmophoria, menstruating women open themselves to the snake deity through sacrifice. Each tears a piglet from a sow, kills it before Snake. To perform these acts, a woman sacrifices her natural nurturing ways. She sacrifices the claims of family, children, village (Burkert 1985, p. 245). She acts out of a vision beyond the habits of caring, beyond the safe structures of society. She places herself outside the demands of civilization and descends to the deity who exists prior to civilization's achievements. She acknowledges that her roots as woman extend to the great below, that life in her body with its natural cycle is sustained by a mystery deep in the underworld. She acknowledges the claim of the underworld deity. She hears her call even in the midst of ordinary life.

In another time, another myth, Holy Inanna, Sumerian Queen of Heaven, hears her call. The myth of the descent of Inanna to the underworld begins like this:

	in great heaven
SHE	turned her ear
	to great earth
	in great heaven
THE GODDESS	turned her ear
	to great earth
	in great heaven
INANNA	turned her ear
	to great earth
	left heaven
MY LADY	abandoned earth
	went down below
	left heaven
INANNA	abandoned earth
	went down below

Inanna enacts a similar mythic pattern to that of the Thesmophoria. Clothed in her seven garments of power, she approaches the realm of her older sister, Ereshkigal, Queen of the Great Below, whose hair tangles on her head like leeks, like writhing snakes. Ereshkigal orders Inanna's garments removed as she passes through the seven underworld gates. Piece by painful piece, Inanna loses the elements of her power, the elements of the achievements of civilization which her garments represent. Naked and bowed low, she approaches the throne of Ereshkigal. For this audacity the judges down below cry out SACRILEGE:

fix on her the death eye
shout at her the wrath words
cry out SACRILEGE

they beat the doomed woman
into a piece of meat
hang her rotting flesh
on a peg

She dies before the power under the ground. Her flesh rots, turns green. After three days and three nights, Inanna's rotting flesh is brought back to life. She climbs out of the chasm accompanied by underworld demons. The demons surround her, cling to her side. They emerge into the upper world with Inanna, incarnate in Inanna, speak through her voice, act through her power.

Inanna is herself the yearly sacrifice in this downgoing and uprising of great antiquity. The demons accompany her uprising just as the rattle of Snake accompanies the Greek women out of the chasm. It is said that the demons who accompany Inanna:

> are never held in the
> sweet legs of a spouse
> tear the spouse
> from the lap of her husband
>
> never kiss a sweet child
> snatch the child from the nurse
> the bride from her wedding bed

The demons, like Snake, rattle and hiss, know nothing of human caring, are ruled by the queen below in whose presence Inanna is transformed.

Before a woman of our time can bring fertility to the field and to herself, before she can realize her creative powers, she must participate in the downgoing. She must gather herself together. She must remove herself from the ongoingness of her daily life. She must descend into the chasm, go deep into the earth, under the ground. She must take with her an offering for that which sustains life, Snake. She must remind herself of her inexorable bond to Snake through her body, renew her bond with a promise. She must give to Snake a little pig, or her valued possessions, or even her life. She must give her sacrifice to the underlying, sustaining mystery and then wait while her gift rots. She is naked now and bowed low. The snakes dance around her and around her gift and are pleased. They eat the rotting flesh. They accept the woman's gift. When the time comes, they bless their bond with the woman, load her baskets with the transformed stinking flesh, send her away. She returns to the upper world with the substance of her own creativity.

The mystery of the Thesmophoria tells us that woman's creativity comes from below. To receive the gift, she must go down. There in the dark dwelling place of primal life, she encounters an older sister, one who lives prior to herself, one who supports the fragile structure of civilization. The encounter shakes her narrow beliefs.

Her beliefs fall before the claim of the primacy of life itself. She returns enlarged, expanded. She returns with gifts of understanding, with praise. On her lips is a song:

Holy Ereshkigal
sweet is your praise
Holy Ereshkigal
sweet is your praise

Holy Ereshkigal
sweet is your praise

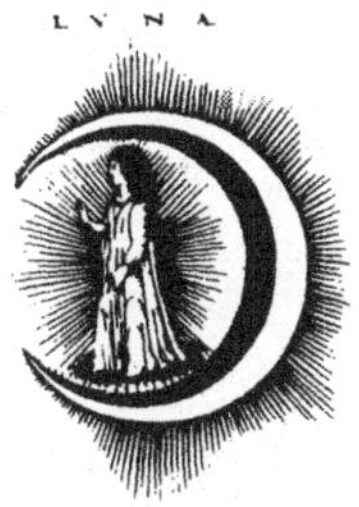

SECTION V

Beyond the Underworld

Into New Life

The woman has survived the ordeal of the underworld and returned from that dark abode to ordinary life. She bears now the marks of the initiation on the inner chambers of her soul where Ereshkigal sits heavily upon her throne. Life in the upper world goes on as before. No one may notice the change in her at all.

The woman feels shaken, raw still where the wounds of her stripping have not healed. She is terrified of what lies ahead. Slowly, slowly new images erupt and spread over her old way of seeing like the changing forms in a kaleidoscope. This is the first hint of the gift Ereshkigal promised. The woman's world is the same, but she begins to see differently. When she left, she was safe in the hands of the fathers and the father god. The initiation wrenched her away from that familiar role, good daughter to the father. Now she wonders who she is, feeling only the dreadful pain of the loss of her former identity and the cleaned-out transparency of one waiting to begin.

The goddess at the center of her universe who most exactly mirrors who she may become is Inanna and Ereshkigal rolled into one. This goddess is the transformed Inanna who, as queen of heaven and earth, balances her authority over the achievements of civilization with her newly acquired underworld powers. The woman, too, while enjoying the comforts of civilization, is beginning to see clearly with Ereshkigal's cutting eye of death, which bores through superficiality, sentimentality, and manipulative self-serving.

This double edge of the transformed goddess is uncharted territory for most of us in modern life. Surviving the underworld passage, the woman now encompasses the full range of femaleness, of the archetypal feminine. On the one hand, she is a raging harpy, vicious, violent, ruthless. On the other, she is full of care and comfort and is the source of creativity. The raw force of the feminine is the side of the goddess that has been banished to the dark of the underworld. This cluster of characteristics, her "dark side," fills the interstices of women's bodies, smoldering in dark blood. She erupts boiling and savage. She is Ereshkigal enraged at her outcast prison. She strikes terror in the heart of the one chosen to carry her into the world.

A raging, vicious woman is likely to be locked up as criminal or mad. Our transformed woman soon finds she must dress Ereshkigal in more-becoming garments. The woman, after all, is not a goddess. She must tap the creative gift she brought from below and invent ways to present her newfound awareness. At this point, sadly, she is alone. There are no ready-made cultural forms or institutions into which Ereshkigal will fit. She must make them up as she goes. Hopefully she will find other travelers on the same road to accompany her on her way.

The poems and essays in this section attempt to describe the transformed Inanna and the woman who lives from that archetypal feminine awareness which the underworld passage kindles. The poems are by the High Priestess Enheduanna who lived in Sumer in 2300 B.C. Devotee of Inanna, she described this goddess in her poetry as Inanna in the fullness of her powers, Inanna transformed by the underworld passage, carrying Ereshkigal in her bones.

Enheduanna is the first person of record to have signed a piece of literature, making her the first poet in the world. Remaining to us are three long poems written to Inanna and a series of forty-two temple hymns. Her position as High Priestess to the Moon God, Nanna, at Ur, was a commanding podium from which to spread her theology. The poems elevate Inanna to a position equal or superior to the traditional great gods of Sumer. Enheduanna must have understood what it means to live from this archetypal feminine base. Sensing the threat that the gods of the spirit raise against the primacy of matter, against nature as the rock-bottom underpinning of the work of the divine, she unseated them and placed Inanna in their stead. This unseating is not unlike what a modern woman has to do in order to return to her roots in the feminine.

The two essays "Uncursing the Dark" and "Forward into the

Past" circumambulate this process of unseating primary loyalty to the fathers in order to uncover feminine roots. The essays echo each other. The first focuses on the historical changeover from a religion based on the primacy of nature to a religion based on the spirit entirely separate from nature. The second essay recounts the long stream of ancestors reaching back into the Paleolithic who worshipped the goddess in all her aspects. These historical events build a foundation for the woman whose descent pulls her into her female roots. They provide a comforting structure for the one who exits from the underworld and sees no place in our current world where she can find support and guidance. The images from these ancient cultures suggest a psychological matrix of life built on the feminine: women's experience was venerated, its passages honored with ritual from birth to death.

Interwoven in the essays are examples of women in all stages of this passage through the underworld and out. These women have been seized by life circumstance or by the compelling force of inner images from dreams or visions or fertile imagination and are able to follow that autonomous attraction we call the unconscious psyche as it tumbles them toward an altogether new orienting matrix, the archetypal feminine. The essays barely hint at the promise this new design may bring. That will unfold only when you, all of you, write your own story.

Excerpts from Poems of the High Priestess Enheduanna

From "The Exaltation of Inanna"

Queen of all given powers
unveiled clear light
unfailing woman wearing brilliance
cherished in heaven and earth

chosen, sanctified in heaven
You
grand in your adornments
crowned with your beloved goodness
rightfully you are High Priestess

your hands seize the seven fixed powers
        my queen of fundamental forces
        guardian of unchanging cosmic sources

you lift up the elements
bind them to your hands
gather in powers
press them to your breast

vicious dragon you spew
        venom poisons the land
like the storm god you howl
        grain wilts on the ground

swollen flood rushing down the mountain
YOU ARE INANNA
SUPREME IN HEAVEN AND EARTH

This rendition of the poems of Enheduanna is by Betty Meador with translations and assistance from Dr. Daniel Foxvog.

From "Inanna and Ebeh"

INANNA! PORTENTOUS ONE!
HOLY! ILL-BODING!
FURY OVERTURNS HER HEART!

with screech of hinge
she flings wide the gate
of the house of battle

her hands pull the bolt lock
on its lapis lazuli door

bedlam unleashed
she sends down a raging battle
hurls a storm from her wide arms
to the ground below

thin sinew the woman strings
for her flawless arrows

and hurricane winds
swift-piercing, stinging
fly with Inanna's fury
suck loosened earth into sweet air
dust chokes every blink and breath
broken bits and fiery chips
swirl in the dust dark air

my Queen batters the mountain[1]
plants her heels hard
rubs dagger's edge on a whet stone

---

[1]Ebeh has been identified as a mountain in southeastern Iraq.

grabs Ebeh by the neck
as she would a sheaf of rushes

in ear-splitting waves
her shrill cries pierce
Ebeh's failing heart

with stones from its own slopes
she pelts she pounds
thud dub thud dub
storms of stones crack its sides
damp and writhing snakes
tangled in branches
drop at her drear bidding
spitting deadly venom

and her tongue's poison
hurls a green-wilting curse
over forest and fruit-bearing trees

she shows no mercy
to its green plant rows
a parching drought she blows
dust dry air in her pitiless wake
gusts over stems of verdant growth
not a moist drop stays

in the bent and withered grass
she strikes fires
flames cut the sky to the boundary stones
flames dance in the smoke stained air
spread at a glance from the queen's glare

holy Inanna
fresh faced, fearless
vigor of a young man commanding

wrestles the mountain to its knees
stands the victor at its base

From "Lady of Largest Heart"

I

with mighty stones she pelts
and the mountain
like a clay pot
crumbles
with her might
she melts the mountain
into a vat of sheepfat

She is Inanna
Bearer of Happiness
whose strapping command
hip-dagger in hand
spreads radiance over the land

fish dragged from the deep
in her stretched-out net
never will slip through
birds trapped in her nimble cast
thrash in the fine-eyed mesh

what she has crushed to powder
never will rise up
the scent of fear stains her robe
she wears
the carved-out ground plan
of heaven and earth

who seeks her word
does not look to AN[2]
the great god assembly
prattles in confusion
cannot fathom her plan's execution
she holds the life of heaven
with her single hand

fierce Lady Wild Cat
sovereign of the Annuna[3]
Inanna
you draw men into unending strife
or crown with fame a favored person's life

II

merely open your mouth
and tables turn
your glance
clogs ears
never to hear
your frown blackens the light of noon

your heart picks the moment of ruin
the place you name trembles

what is yours
cannot be crushed

who dares oppose
your deeds
Queen of heaven and earth

---

[2]God of heaven
[3]Council of the gods.

no bribes sway
divine verdicts you say
Inanna
judge of the palace throng

more weighty than a mountain
is an oath sworn in your name
AN cannot compete

when you heed your nimble wit
all the gods around
cast their joyless faces down
you alone are glorious

all gods
all heaven and earth
call you
Great Mother Cow

scarcely lift your eyes
the gods
open mouthed
attend

in your dwelling
the great gods stand
saying sweet prayers

and praise
your dreadful brilliance
gladly live
at your lofty breast

no sanctions cease unending praise
where is your single name
not glorious

Uncursing the Dark

Restoring the Lost Feminine

"Eleanor Roosevelt said it is better to light a single candle than to curse the darkness. I say I would rather uncurse the dark."

Poet Judy Grahn (1988)

I have taken the theme of this conference[1] as an opportunity to examine our culture's strong bias against the dark. My pursuit rose out of a conviction that women are by their instinctual nature at home in the dark, that women's natural way of transformation out of an ordered, civilized society is down into the dark, and that a female-based religion would include as a natural part of its worship the powers of the dark.

If my convictions have any truth in them, then women in our culture are separated from the pathways of their natural growth. Adapted to a religion of light and a culture that upholds light and reason, women are cut off from their roots and from their creative transformative energies which lie in the chaos and mystery of the dark.

The framework of culture has such a binding effect that nature's instinctual pull can be held in bondage to the consensual perceptions and beliefs of a society. We are learning this fact ever more clearly from the work of anthropologists as well as psychologists. Anthropologists describe how the little Manu grows into the big Manu, the little Navajo grows into the big Navajo, even the little Texan grows into the big Texan. The subtleties of a culture's style as well as its content mold the growing child.

Reprinted from *Quadrant: The Journal of Contemporary Jungian Thought* (1989, vol. 22, no. 1, p. 27), courtesy of the C. G. Jung Foundation for Analytical Psychology of New York.

[1]National Conference of Jungian Analysts, Chicago, September 1987, "The Influence of American Culture on Analysis."

Psychologists consider the effect of culture on the individual. Daniel Stern, in his book on self formation in infancy, says, "Events at a societal level make an issue more salient for the mother–infant dyad" (1985, p. 23). Socializing pressures are largely culturally determined. The terrible twos are not terrible in all societies, he says, but have become terrible in our culture because of socializing pressures that clash with the child's developmental leaps at this age. Thus the child is molded psychologically, sometimes even physically as in circumcision or head shaping, to fit the perceptions of beauty, order, and goodness of the larger society.

The making of culture is part of what humans do to organize the experience of living in a group. Joseph Henderson's work on the influence of the cultural unconscious, and specifically on the four cultural attitudes in individuals—the social, the religious, the aesthetic, and the philosophic—has been an invaluable help in understanding the shaping role of culture. His discussion of the religious attitude clarifies the basis of our cultural viewpoint toward the dark:

> There is, however, a cultural difference in religious attitude between people who start from an original monotheism and those whose religion is primarily polytheistic. (1984, p. 29)

Monotheistic belief moves decisively away from the dark, while polytheism contains the dark and light within its belief system. These two contrasting systems powerfully affect the traditions and values of the cultures built around them. Henderson contrasts the two in their attitude toward death and toward transcendence:

> The religious experience of death is the same for all, a universal "dark night of the soul," but the renewal which follows it may take two very different roads toward enlightenment: the monotheistic, basically patriarchal, religions favor the image of a resurrection, while polytheism favors the conception of rebirth, with its matriarchal coloring. The first is linear (historically understood) and transcendent which really means "final." The second is recurrent, like the eons or the seasons, and is conceived as cyclic rather than linear—Mircea Eliade's "eternal recurrence of all things." (1984, pp. 29-30)

Henderson says the initiatory rites of the two express their basic difference. In polytheism, the rites take place down in the underground or in a courtyard. The god image "is a symbol of emergence and growth taking place within it like a plant growing in a well-cultivated garden" (Henderson 1984, p. 30). In monotheism, the initiation "is conceived as 'a journey,' a mystical approach to the godhead leading to spiritual perfection, a sort of 'pilgrim's progress'" (ibid., p. 30). Polytheistic transformation takes place down in the dark of the underworld or in the containing rectangle of the courtyard, while monotheistic transformation takes place in the linear journey toward the light.

Our own American culture, built on Judeo-Christian monotheism, carries a strong bias against the dark, against chaos, the dark side of order, against the cyclic which includes waxing and waning, against the feminine as it is related to the dark, and ultimately against the containing of opposites in favor of the light only. I want to examine this bias, which I see as an archetypal perception, galvanized into a religion, and filtered into our bones as truth.

It is difficult to pinpoint the exact origin of this bias against the dark. I will begin with an examination of the creation story in Genesis because it contains a cursing of the serpent, that ambiguous, emotionally charged creature associated with dark powers. Genesis also contains an order for the subjugation of woman. As the traditional starting point of our cultural history, the story warrants a closer look.

In the Genesis story, we meet a god who prefers paradise for his creation. He prefers that the man and woman he created remain in the abundance of the garden, ignorant of the world outside. He goes to extremes to keep the couple from knowledge of that surrounding world, telling them they will die if they eat of a certain forbidden tree. The serpent reveals this god's deceit. The serpent says the couple will not die if they eat from the tree but will be like god, knowing good and evil.

When the couple and the serpent go against the god's wishes, they are punished. Because Adam listens to his wife and eats the fruit, this god, Yahweh, curses the ground he must till. Because Eve disobeys, Yahweh multiplies her pain in childbearing and sets her husband to rule over her. But the most interesting punishment for our purpose is Yahweh's curse of the serpent. The account says that Yahweh puts enmity between the serpent and the woman. Why does the story make such a point of this? Why not simply curse the serpent to crawl on her belly? What *was* the relation between the serpent and woman?

One does not have to look far to find that the serpent is the symbol of the deity at the very heart of the ancient goddess-dominated polytheistic religions. The worship of snake as deity reaches far back into the Upper Paleolithic, where it appears in meander and spiral patterns. In Neolithic Old Europe and Mesopotamia, snake deities wind on the body of the goddess, or she has a snake head and nurses a snake baby. In ancient Greece, the snake deities were central to the earth religions. Jane Ellen Harrison says the earth-born goddesses were all originally snakes (1962, p. 260). In the women's ritual of the Thesmophoria, which later developed into the Eleusinian mysteries, the participants descended into a deep chasm to feed the snake deities. Thus, for the religions of Greece, Old Europe, and the ancient Near East, the snake was a primary image of the deity. Sometimes the snake was sexless; more often she was female. She was the nonhuman sister who lived in the primordial mystery of the dark.

In the Thesmophoria ritual in Greece, women carried baby pigs into a chasm, slit their bellies open, and fed them to the snake deities. That portion of the flesh which the snake did not eat rotted, and the women carried the putrid flesh out of the chasm, mixed it with seed, and placed it on the altar to be blessed for planting.

On the second day of the ritual, the women fasted, sitting on the ground. Since in preparation for the ritual the women had drunk a potion to bring on menstruation, they bled on this fasting day into the field. On the third and final day, the women planted the seeds with rejoicing ("The Thesmophoria: A Women's Ritual," pp. 92–103).

Two aspects of this ritual help us understand women's relationship to snake, the pig sacrifice, and the requisite menstruation. In eating the flesh of baby pigs, the snake deity asserts her primacy over the piglet, a household animal so like a human baby. Symbolically, the women sacrifice human caring, relatedness, and nurturing to the larger reality of the impersonal being represented by the snake. Snake represents what IS, the givenness of the natural world which cannot be changed, being itself, the autonomous life force moving through our bodies and through the natural world. In this regard, menstruation belongs to snake, as the cycle moves through women's bodies autonomously and gives forth its fertile blood.

The wisdom of the ancient polytheistic goddess-oriented religions rests on the facts of the natural world. This wisdom tempers love, nurturing, and relatedness with a grounding in impersonal reality. Bearing these opposites, both natural, instinctual nurturing and the equally natural awe and submission to impersonal reality is the implicit wisdom of a transformation down into the dark. The myths and rituals of descent, such as the myth of Inanna's descent to the underworld or the ritual of the Thesmophoria or of the Villa of Mysteries of Pompeii, are rites that pertain to women; the ancient wisdom they express is women's wisdom.

When Yahweh placed enmity between the woman and the snake, he separated woman from her powerful alliance with and understanding of the dark chthonic world of impersonal reality, a separation still operating in American culture today. Yahweh tried to create a world of goodness and plenty, tried by his powerful will and deceit to hold the humans there, fashioning for them a false sense of what is. His way of punishing them for their disobedience was to expel them from Paradise into the natural world of the opposites.

The creation story in Genesis stands at the end of thousands of years of polytheistic religions. The sacred images of the deity in the Paleolithic and Neolithic were predominantly female. Abundant archeological finds in the ancient Near East, in Anatolia, and in Old Europe tell the story of stable, highly developed cultures whose life was based on the sacred female deities in both dark and light aspects. These cultures are our direct ancestors, and they contain the dark that Yahweh banished. Following are some examples of images from the Neolithic cultures which contain dark and light.

The culture at Çatal Hüyük on the Anatolian plain lasted from 6700 to 5700 B.C. At its height Çatal Hüyük held a population of ten thousand people. Many of the rooms in the apartmentlike structures at this site are elaborately decorated shrines. On one wall might be a large sculpture of the goddess giving birth, or pregnant, or paired with her maiden daughter with, on an adjoining wall, exquisite paintings of the huge black vultures in the act of excarnation. The dead of Çatal Hüyük were placed away from the village on the plain, and the vultures stripped the body of flesh in about twenty minutes. The bones were then gathered and buried under the sleeping platforms of the houses. In these shrines, life and death were celebrated simultaneously. Nurturing and devouring are depicted together as well in the many breasts molded on the walls of the shrines from whose nipples protrude beaks of vultures, "lower jaws of wild boar, heads of weasel and fox, all scavengers and harbingers of death" (Mellaart 1970, p. 312).

A later culture, called Old Europe by Marija Gimbutas, stretched from the Black Sea to the Adriatic, reaching its zenith around 5000 B.C. For several thousand years the culture revolved around its religious core, the worship of goddesses. Some 30,000 sculptures have been excavated from 3,000 sites, unique representations of a goddess in two primary aspects. One is the goddess as giver

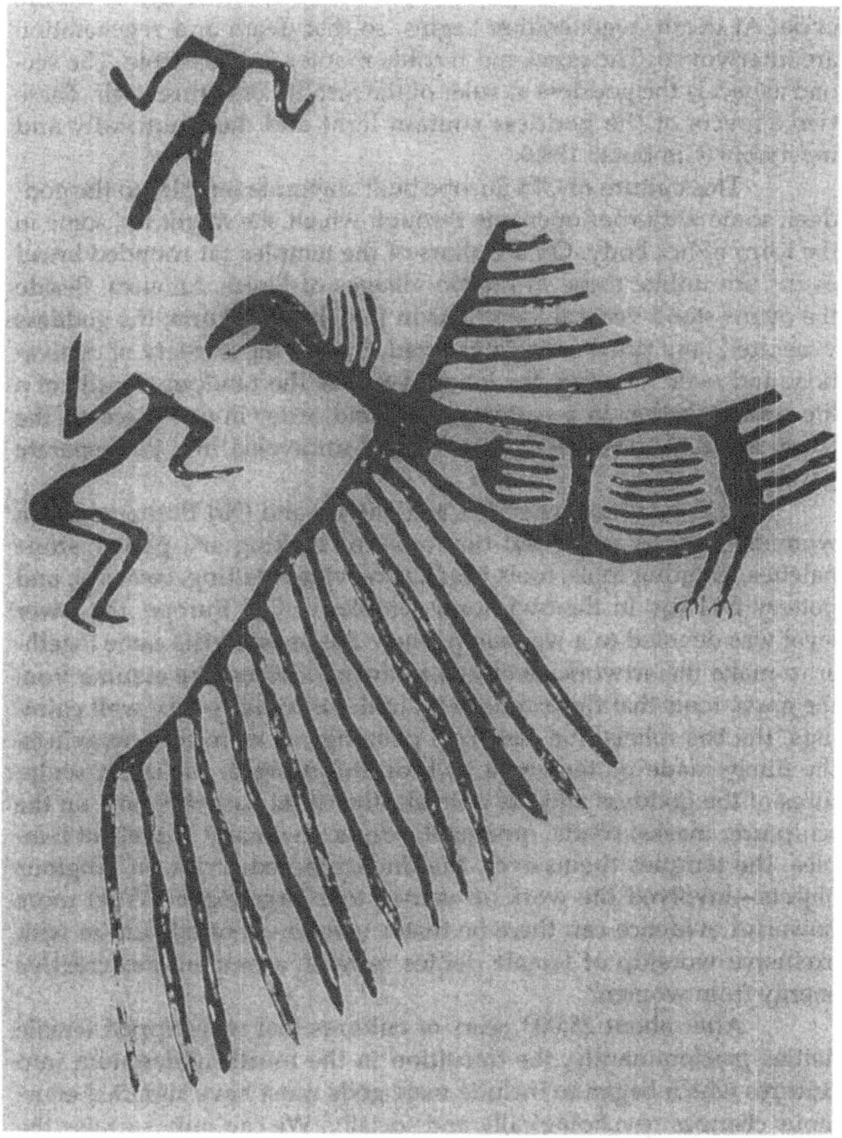

Figure 4. Vulture attacking two humans, one of whom is crouched in the posture of the dead. From a Çatal Hüyük shrine (from Mellaart 1967, p. 93).

of both life and death. In this aspect, she controls the length of the life cycle. At death, regeneration begins, so that death and regeneration are interwoven. The good and terrible mother is indivisible. The second aspect is the goddess as ruler of the fertility of nature itself. These two aspects of the goddess contain light and dark naturally and inevitably (Gimbutas 1982).

This culture of Old Europe built elaborate temples to the goddess, some with roof openings through which she might fly, some in the form of her body. On the altars of the temples sat rounded bread ovens not unlike those in Pueblo villages of North America. Beside the ovens stood vertical looms. As in the Thesmophoria, the goddess venerated here ruled over daily bread, fruit of the mystery of cultivation, and over weaving, the loom of fate as the random threads of a life come together in a pattern, chaos and order in one piece on the loom, artfully woven and just as easily unraveled into its disparate parts.

In the cultures of both Çatal Hüyük and Old Europe, only in women's graves are found the tools for making art: paints, stone palettes, painting tools, tools used in weaving, matting, basketry, and pottery making. In the two-storey temples of Old Europe, the lower level was devoted to a workshop where the finest artists came together to make the artwork dedicated to the goddesses. We assume from the grave tools that the exquisite art of these cultures—the wall paintings, the bas reliefs, the elaborate paintings of kilim-type weavings, the finely made pottery with its beautiful designs, the many sculptures of the goddess and her animals, the ritual paraphernalia on the sculpture, masks, beads, ornaments, dress, the many models of temples, the temples themselves, the undeciphered script on religious objects—involved the work of women to a large extent. What more powerful evidence can there be that a woman-centered culture with exclusive worship of female deities releases a tremendous creative energy from women?

After about 25,000 years of cultures that worshipped female deities predominantly, the transition in the fourth millennium into cultures which began to include male gods must have signified enormous changes psychologically and socially. We can only surmise the causes of this transition, but by the time of recorded history male rule of the growing city-states was well in place, and the worship of male deities equaled the worship of female.

We have one piece of evidence, from the Sumerian civilization of southern Mesopotamia, of the difficult conflict between the old religion, in which the goddess contains the cyclic opposites of nature, and the startling new idea, which intrigued the male gods, that nature could be one-sided, bountiful only. The evidence is in a little-known poem by the high priestess, Enheduanna, the first religious head of a united Sumer, and the world's first poet of record. While we may have difficulty recovering the historical events that led to male domination, we can deduce from this poem the psychological impact of the transition.

Enheduanna was a poet, priestess, dream interpreter, and the first high priestess in a line of women who led Sumerian religious life for five hundred years. Her mother may have been Sumerian, but her father was Akkadian from the north. He, King Sargon, was the first to unite northern and southern Mesopotamia, around 2300 B.C. Indeed, Sargon's armies conquered most of the known world.

Enheduanna was a devotee of Inanna. In the three long poems to Inanna which remain to us, she puts forth her understanding of the process of transformation as well as her theology of the feminine. The poem that most explicitly pits feminine against masculine is called "Inanna and Ebeh." In it, Enheduanna tells of a conflict between Inanna and the ruling sky god, An. Their friction focuses on a mountain called Ebeh, a veritable paradise like Eden, where plants, trees, and animals flourish in unending abundance. Inanna is enraged at Ebeh's hubris and grandiosity in claiming to be abundant only. She sets out to destroy the place that will not bow down to her rule, the rule of nature's ebb and flow. An, on the other hand, trembles with fear, and perhaps excitement, that this daring mountain would defy the dark, entangling, thwarting, cyclic demands of the goddess. He will not join Inanna in her confrontation of Ebeh. When An refuses to help her, Inanna hurls her entire arsenal against Ebeh, weapons, fires, storms, even stones from the slopes of the mountain itself. She brings the mountain to its knees.

An, like Yahweh, is taken with the idea of paradise, of the eternal abundance Ebeh seems to enjoy. An trembles with fear before Mt. Ebeh's daring defiance of Inanna. Yahweh, a millennium later, strikes fear in the hearts of Adam and Eve lest they see beyond the good-mother garden into the whole of reality. Both An and Yahweh support a new ideal, one of goodness and unending abundance, which necessarily excludes the feminine domain of death and life, mystery and clarity, chaos and order, dark and light.

An's fascination with and near adoration of Ebeh has the emotional quality of the experience of the anima. The promise of the idealized feminine enabled men, and perhaps women, to imagine worlds beyond the confines of nature. This leap of the imagination was indeed an entirely new possibility of consciousness. The concept of a unifying deity independent of the cycles of the natural world and existing beyond nature and matter is the basis of monotheism. Did this concept grow out of a split in the archetype of the feminine between dark and light? M. T. Colonna, in her article on Lilith, makes this point:

> Mankind, involved in the conflict between immanence and transcendence, between matter and spirit, suffers the necessity of transcending the side that Lilith offers him, contrasted as it is with his metaphysical side. He experiences the necessity of making a sacrifice to the gods. What, then, should be sacrificed, if not this carnal side? At this point the anima differentiates itself. (1980, p. 341)

The story of Inanna and Ebeh from 2300 B.C. is clearly a precursor to the Garden of Eden story in Genesis. Indeed, *edin* is a Sumerian word denoting the wild lands outside the cities, and archeologist Juris Zarins believes he has located the actual Garden of Eden in the very heart of Sumer at the confluence of the Tigris and Euphrates near the Persian Gulf (Hamblin 1987, p. 127). Now we can see the Genesis creation story as the culmination of a developmental attempt on the part of the masculine to eliminate the impersonal, natural power of snake and her dark realm.

The two stories, Ebeh and Eden, have different endings. In Enheduanna's story of Ebeh, Inanna in the full force of her power throws herself against the mountain and destroys it, demolishing at the same time An's hopes for a paradise on earth. Here is what she says to Ebeh after her victory:

> MOUNTAIN! she cries
> EBEH!
>
> because you puff yourself up
> because you stand so high
> dress up so beautiful
> make yourself so green and luscious
> put on a royal robe
> stretch your hand straight to An
>
> do not wipe your nose on the ground
> do not flatten your lips in the dust
> I HAVE KILLED YOU!
> I HAVE STRUCK YOUR HEART WITH SORROW!

you thick hided elephant
I will twist your trunk

you oversized bull
I will wrench your neck
grab your thick horns
throw you in the dust
stomp you with my hatred
grind my knees in your neck
till tears wet your face
sorrow grips your heart

TURN YOUR BACK ON ME !
may the bleak bird of heartbreak
nest in your shadows

In this poem, two archetypal thrusts vie for dominance. Inanna, on one side, carries the fullness of the archetypal feminine. She demands that we face and accept her rule, which brings disaster, anguish, tragedy, and death into our lives as readily as it brings goodness and plenty. No one is excepted. We cannot hide behind the narcissistic attitude "It won't happen to me" or expect to bargain using good behavior. Inanna demands that we bow down, become submissive to her as giver of our fate. If we are fully open to her, we cannot avoid the suffering and tragedy that is woven into life. Inanna is not evil. She is the stark horror and beauty of what is. To open to her is to stretch oneself between the opposites. An, on the other hand, carries a rather one-sided aspect of the masculine. He is fascinated with the possibility of perpetual ease and abundance. He longs for the land of Ebeh where adversity does not exist. He is even intimidated by the promise of paradise and refuses to support Inanna in her fury against Ebeh's pride. An's attitude underlies that of the hero whose goal is victory over the monstrous dark. In his later incarnation as Yahweh, he brands the dark as evil. Eventually this patriarchal attitude of privilege, mastery, and conquest gained dominance in our cultural history.

The serpent goddess in Eden does not rise in Eve's defense. Her power had diminished in the thousand years between the two stories. In that same thousand years, the advances women had made psychologically in understanding their nature, in understanding the process of transformation, in understanding their roots in the primordial dark, were all lost. Enheduanna's poetry lay buried until this century, as did women's fine achievements in the great civilizations of Anatolia, Mesopotamia, and Old Europe. It appears that full realization of the heroic masculine could come about only through the subjugation of women and the elimination of their religion and through the split in the archetypal feminine between the dark and the light.

American culture is part of the tradition that strives to overcome the dark. In its bias against the dark, American culture, like all cultures in the West, rests on the Judaic creation story in which living in full reality is a punishment. Yahweh banishes Adam and Eve into hardship and suffering, into the real world, the same real world of opposites that Inanna embraces as the poignant dark and light of her domain, the very essence of the feminine. Inanna insists we see the opposites as a divine gift, while Yahweh holds out the tantalizing possibility that life could have been different.

I believe we are once again in a period of enormous transition equal to that which took place around 3500 B.C. The change comes from a new emergence of the archetypal feminine in her dark and light fullness. Colonna cites the renewal of interest in Lilith as testimony "to the rebirth of the mythologem in human consciousness" (1980, p. 332):

> We could, however, postulate a "new consciousness" yet more advanced than the patriarchal, emerging out of the union of both matriarchal and patriarchal elements . . . . It seems, then, that the myth of Lilith suggests a way to break the fixation with "being below," repressed and maltreated, and there seems to be an analogy here with the lunar, matriarchal spirit that seeks to be accepted into the realm of consciousness. (1980, p. 336)

Freudians talk about the split-off feminine in a different language from Jungians. Winnicott describes the female element as the experience of being and the male element as that of doing. Using Winnicott's terms, Guntrip makes this statement in discussing repression, withdrawal, and dissociation:

> It appears to me that clinically *it is always the female element that we find dissociated in both men and women, and that the fundamental dissociation is of the female element.* (1968, p. 254)

I would say that the dissociation of the female element is a cultural phenomenon acquired through three thousand years of primacy of the patriarchal gods. In the archetypal pattern of the unconscious in our culture, the god An still trembles in terror in the face of the powerful, all-giving mother who holds men in the grip of the mother complex. The god Yahweh rages at the disobedient woman and curses the dark reaches of the feminine, binding women to the demanding norms of the culture and to the negative animus. Little wonder the female element is dissociated.

Feminist writers have struggled with Freud's description of the basic complexes in men and women. Recent works by feminist psychoanalysts expand Freud's late revision of the Oedipus complex in relation to little girls (Irigaray 1985a, 1985b). Freud had to acknowledge in his late writing the persistence into adult life of the preoedipal attachment between mother and girl child, an attachment based on an experience of female body to like female body (Freud 1920, 1931, p. 227). It is this attachment that forms the basis of a theory which rescues women from the erroneous definition of them under the Oedipus complex as suffering from penis envy. The girl child's experience of and attachment to the mother's body, I believe, relates to her experience of the archetypal Self as female. Jacqueline Rose states the Freudian feminist position thus:

> The privileged relationship of women to that [female] origin gives them access to an archaic form of expressivity outside the circuit of linguistic exchange. This point of origin is the maternal body, an undifferentiated space and yet one in which the girl child recognizes herself. The girl then has to suppress or devalue that fullness of recognition in order to line up within the order of the phallic term. (Rose 1986, p. 78)

The girl child has an initial anatomical connection to the feminine. In Freudian terms, she has access "to an archaic form of expressivity," Jung's experience of the archetypes. Here she recognizes herself, experiencing a fullness of recognition in her relationship to the mother. This fullness of recognition she must either "suppress or devalue" in order to live out the "phallic term," that is, the masculine definition of woman.

As analysts we are given the task, I believe, of fostering the retrieval in women of that full recognition of themselves in the archetypal feminine. We must correct for the phallic definition of women prevalent in our culture, a definition that requires women to suppress or devalue their own female nature. Recognition of the archetypal feminine involves educating ourselves to its full expression.

For most women, experiencing the fullness of recognition in the feminine is a new experience. A full woman, she gives up her favored status as father's daughter and helpmate to her husband and stands in her stature and strength as a woman, restoring her identification with the mother, with the feminine, and with women. She becomes a woman-identified woman.

This transition from the acceptable adaptation she has made in a masculine-defined culture to the recognition of the fullness of herself in relation to the archetypal feminine is a transition of enormous proportions. She is switching religions. She is betraying the fathers. She is aligning herself with the outcasts. She is returning to an affirmation of the dark. No easy task, this transition may take years or a lifetime. There is no doubt, however, that many women are confronted by powerful unconscious images pulling in this direction.

The transition happens primarily to women in midlife. The call of Inanna into the underworld comes in the form of a movement inside, a tremor a woman "hears." It comes after her successful adaptation in the world. Inanna is married, not a virgin, a matron, not a puella. The modern woman has built a substantial self which works in the outer world, which has been shaped by civilization to its mold. But parallel to the culture's shaping of a self is the lack, the want, the hole inside under which lies the dark primordial feminine, the banished Lilith. The descent into the dark means a shattering of her upper world adaptation. The woman's task is the reintegration of the feminine which has been held below. Nor Hall says of the women pictured in the initiation at the Villa of Mysteries:

> . . . women who are about to go under because they are about to give birth. Women in whom the fruit is seven months ripe, in whom a child is fully formed. These are "expectant" women who are already far into the process of creating some new thing, who know about the submission, the "putting under" of conscious control that happens in labor when the movement from stage to stage is set by some director other than yourself. (Hall 1988, p. 34)

In analysis, the early dreams relating to this theme are usually of the woman's recognition of her status as an alien in someone else's system. She dreams she is in bondage to a con artist or a criminal, or she is a captive to her tyrannical, animus-possessed mother. One woman dreamed she belonged to a group of women who do not believe in the moon. Finding shelter with those who do not believe in the moon cuts a woman off from a full experience of her natural periodicity. Return to a self grounded in periodicity is the rock bottom of female identification. Dreams of menstrual blood also call for this reorientation to the cyclic.

The second period of analysis focuses on the structure of the woman's personal adaptation. Dreams in this period are of cataclysmic destruction of the old order. Patterns that have given her shelter and comfort in the past are being destroyed, sometimes by nuclear disaster, sometimes by natural forces, an uncanny wind or storm, fire or water. Her dreams bring an experience of the chaos of the dark. Doris Lessing's novel, *Memoirs of a Survivor,* vividly describes a woman's passage through this stage. In Lessing's novel, the government of a country is collapsing, and the main character spends her time waiting in the silent rooms of her house, interrupted only by the opening of a mysterious passage through a certain wall into the chaotic mess of her past and steamy scenes from her childhood (Lessing 1975). In analysis, this is a time of painful confrontation with childhood memories. The old order has tumbled in a heap, and picking one's way through the ruins seems a necessary part of laying it to rest.

Women are usually defended against the dark constricting realities of their fates and limitations. Recovery of the memories of damage and evil in their pasts is slow and painful. Ultimately that recovery includes the dark archetypal feminine. Hall describes the initiates as

> these deep weavers who weave tissue to bone out of the substance of their bodies. They too are resistant. Even though they approach the threshold with dignity . . . , they turn in terror when the thunder begins to rumble, knowing that the bull-roarer's simulation of thunder announces an inevitable bolt that will shock and sear Semele, sending her on to that final stage of transformation where what was bound inside is freed. (Hall 1988, p. 34)

These two periods I am describing seldom follow in orderly sequence, but they are identifiable themes and parts of a whole. At some point the goddess herself appears, often during the time of waiting in seemingly meaningless deprivation and despair. Images of her come in dreams. She is a group of hungry hags in the molten center of the earth. She is a black woman who arrives to make love to the dreamer. She is a trollop, a whore; she is uncouth, brassy, cheap. She is a priestess leading an initiation in a room of fire. She is seductive, desiring the dreamer, awakening in her erotic love for a woman. She is a spring which wells up unexpectedly. She is animal. She is a long-buried pig being dug up. She is a wild cat feeding her young on a woman's lap.

She often appears angry, enraged at being so neglected. She

often comes in a form our culture defines as outcast. She is often too much to take, asking the woman to do something terribly difficult, way out of the bounds of her ordinary life. She often forces the dreamer to face the harsh realities of death, suffering, loss, meaninglessness. She sometimes pushes the woman to the brink of madness. She places her gift of the dark truth on the altar for worship. In all her guises, she introduces the dreamer to a new order.

Is this process I have described different from any analysis which goes through the breakup of the old adaptation in favor of a larger encompassing of the psyche? The difference is in the feminine images of the Self emerging from the unconscious and in our recognition of these images as a call to a new order. Colonna says, "The Western woman of today searches to re-grasp religious, mythical and ancestral grounds for her psychological and moral emargination and of her 'guilt' or 'fault'" (1980, p. 326). Women are being challenged by these ancient images to accept nothing less than a reorientation of the psyche away from Yahweh's curse to a new experience of Inanna's full incarnation. Women are being challenged to stretch themselves beyond the security and familiarity of American cultural roles, into a new embrace of dark and light. Women are being asked to invent new cultural forms which will enhance and contain the whole expression of the female Self and to pioneer in the face of stiff opposition outside and their own fears, doubts, and loneliness inside.

As analysts we must set aside our cultural biases, listen carefully as the unconscious presents a new way for women. We have to be willing to uncurse the dark, to look into the face of the dark with expectation and humility. Out of the dark, women will restore their natural wholeness. Having been banished for 3,000 years from the doorstep of their own religion, women are entering a new sanctuary of self-understanding that will grow out of repeated descents into the fertile dark of the imagination. Out of the dark, new cultural forms will take life. The burden of consciousness these women bear will carry us into the new age.

Forward into the Past

Reemergence of the Archetypal Feminine

The north Texas town where I was born is situated just across the Red River from what then were the Indian lands of Oklahoma. The town sits on another frontier, between the rich farming territories of east Texas, where the culture is more akin to the Deep South, and the vast plains, ranchlands, and oil strikes of west Texas, whose culture is typified by a wild and hearty freedom.

My parents were upward striving. My mother had been a schoolteacher in Tennessee and married late for that era. She was nearly thirty. My father was born in the French settlement of Paris, Texas, and although uneducated, he became a successful businessman. I was the second of three children. When I was one year old, we moved to the brick house that our family was to inhabit the rest of my parents' lives. The house was in a new, placid neighborhood on the edge of town. An old dairy across the street had been turned into a residence, and I spent hours in my childhood around the now-landscaped pond where the cows once drank water.

In those mid-Depression days my parents somehow managed to have a housekeeper. We called her our "nurse-girl." These women were a welcome refuge for me from my mother's anxiety about appearance and form. One of these women I remember in particular, Elizabeth Trimm.

Liz was, in my mother's words, "a big-boned, good German girl," from a nearby predominately German community. My mother meant that Liz could work hard for long hours without tiring and was not so attractive that she would have suitors to bother us. My parents paid her $5.00 a week.

Liz had been raised in an orphanage and told wonderful, harrowing tales of her life with the other orphan children. She taught me to thread a needle, to tie a single- or double-strand knot. She could

---

Based on "Forward into the Past" in *Dreams in Analysis,* Nathan Schwartz-Salant and Murray Stein, editors. © 1990 by Chiron Publications.

wring water out of the doll clothes I washed until they were nearly dry, twisting the little dresses with her rough, strong hands.

She also taught me a divining method using a Bible and a key, wringing the mystery of the feminine out of that awesome, dry book so dear to my father. We would sit on the steps outside the back door. Liz inserted a skeleton key into the pages of the Bible so that it lay right on the passage in the book of Ruth, where Ruth speaks to Naomi these words:

> Entreat me not to leave thee or to return from following after thee; for whither thou goest, I will go, and whither thou lodgest, I will lodge; thy people shall be my people, and thy God, my God. (1, 16)

Liz would then close the Bible on the key, tie a scarf around the Bible like a sling, cross it around the protruding handle of the key, and tie it so that Bible and key were snugly secured together.

Now came the divining. With her fingers pinching the top of the key, Liz turned the key slowly so that its head, tucked between the pages of the Bible, wedged the book open slightly. I placed my index finger under one side of the sticking-out oval top of the key, and she placed her index finger under the other side. Carefully, we let the Bible-key-scarf contraption dangle between us. One of us would have asked a question, burning, important questions like, "Does Sydney Wagghorn (my third grade idol) like me?" Or Liz would ask, "Will Billy Piper ask me out?" Or I might ask, "Will I get a bicycle for Christmas?" Then we would repeat together the sacred words from Ruth, "Entreat me not to leave thee. . . ."

If the precariously wedged key held its place, the answer to our question was "NO." If, however, the key moved flat again between the pages, as it was, of course, more likely to do as the weight of the Bible swung under our fingers, then the book would turn, slowly and mysteriously, bringing the blessed answer from the universe, "YES!" How many magical hours we spent on the back steps with Bible, scarf, and key, probing the One-who-knows-all-things for answers.

Liz was a good mother to me with her earthy practicality. More important, out of her somewhat unsocialized orphan past, she brought to me a glimpse of the hidden world of the feminine. She knew ways other than logic and reason to tease out the truth. She knew intuitive mysterious ways to connect us to an underlying knowing. There on the back steps, we huddled together beyond the bounds of parental culture. We traveled back in time to that remnant of woman's devotion to woman in the book of Ruth and to hints of a female world beyond imagining in this little Texas town.

The mystery Liz tapped touched a responsive chord in me. I now realize she lived from the feminine, which had not been erased in her by the orphanage world or by the German peasant farm culture from which she came. Our divining derived from our direct female heritage of the dark mysteries of ancient priestesses or seers or witches. Even now I can feel the warm opening inside which occurred when we sat over our speaking Bible. I felt an expectant excitement at the hint of worlds beyond the strict confines of Protestant Christianity, worlds I was drawn to and longed to inhabit. Liz carried something which my own mother was missing.

II

In this paper I want to explore the possibility that this vast world of the feminine, with its particular worldview which informs beliefs and actions, with its distinctive forms of initiation and transformation, with its intense bonding between and among women, is largely unknown to us but lies waiting in the psyches of women and appears regularly in women's dreams as a call to individuation along a path we, as a culture, have long since abandoned. This world of the feminine opens in the imagination from a basic core experience of primary relationship to the archetypal feminine.

The idea that a woman's development might rest more authentically on the historical and archetypal matrix of the feminine strongly challenges the Freudian view of the desired female attitude in which the girl in the oedipal phase attaches to her father as love object and experiences her lack of a penis as a deformity. Modern women psychoanalysts have criticized Freud's paradigm and offered in its stead a pattern of female development that is based on a girl's preoedipal attachment to the mother, a pattern which, they assert, also leads to a woman's healthy autonomous maturity (Irigaray 1985).

Euro-American women's experience of being second-class citizens by birth may be, in the Freudian sense, an experience of a loss. While the loss or lack may not be a conscious wish for a penis, it is experienced in the countless ways limits are placed on the woman in the culture. Something is missing. The woman feels deprived. In analysis, she names her deprivation, and we analysts concur, "mother did not give me enough"— enough attention, enough nurturing, enough appreciation, enough understanding. However, underlying

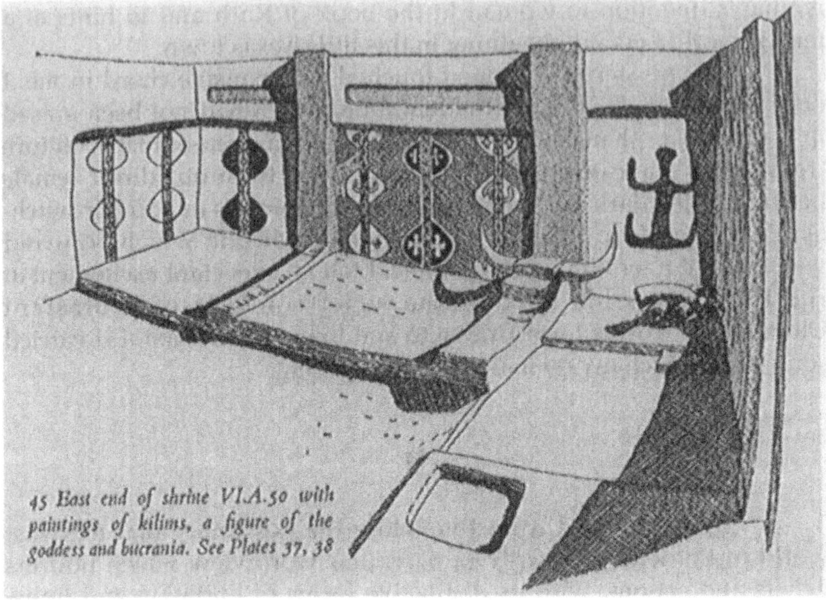

Figure 5. Shrine from Çatal Hüyük with goddess in birth-giving posture and kilim patterns on the walls (from Mellaart 1967, p. 155).

the woman's personal experience of deprivation is another, larger loss. What the mother is missing, and what the culture is missing, is the support of the fully realized power of the archetypal feminine. The lack the woman experiences is not the missing penis. The lack is the absence of the vital symbols of the feminine and its sacred vulva.

III

These feminist psychoanalytic writings emerged during women's recent struggle for redefinition. Synchronistically, archeologists' discoveries in the last three decades have unearthed Neolithic cultures that were oriented toward and sustained by female deities. Offering women historical examples of a feminine-based orientation and identification, these recent Neolithic discoveries call for a serious reconsideration of Freud's views.

As we interpret the remains of these cultures, two facts stand out. Women in these cultures had their own gender-appropriate place and time. The shrines and temples were women's places. The cyclic ritual was women's time.

All the evidence points to women being the priestesses of the worship in the elaborate temples and shrine rooms of these cultures. Here women had place, a specifically set apart place which held, welcomed, and nourished them. This female place was central to the ongoing life of the community. In the sacred place, worship was in the service of the goddess, who reflected perfectly the women's bodies and cyclic development.

Moreover, women had time set apart—a cyclic round of ritually designated time. Great rituals came to pass at the transition points of the seasons. This was women's time based on a science whose timekeeper was the moon. The surge of the menstrual tides in her body matched the waxing and waning of the moon and matched the coming and going of the seasons. Indeed, some of the great rituals required that all the women be menstruating simultaneously; it is likely that they were anyway, living in the close proximity of village life. For these rituals, women whose menses did not synchronize naturally drank an herbal potion to bring on the flow (see p. 95).

Having place and time, women gave birth quite naturally to artistic modes of expression of their creative imagination. The exquisite and varied art forms reflect the artists' imaginative expression of the archetypal feminine.

Surely it is synchronistic that the great Neolithic cultures oriented toward the feminine have been discovered just at the time that the consciousness of women began reaching for autonomous expression. The earliest discoveries coincided with the beginnings of the women's movement in the late nineteenth century, but the major Neolithic discoveries came at the same time as the second wave of the women's movement since World War II. The impact of the discoveries did not hit the scientific world until after C. G. Jung's death, so that the full complexity of the archetype as expressed in the Neolithic could not have been taken into account by Jung. The scope and duration of these ancient cultures is astonishing. Those in Anatolia, the ancient Near East, and Old Europe lie in a continuous line leading to Western civilization, and these are our immediate ancestors. In all of these cultures, figures of the divine female among the artifacts far outnumber figures of males. These societies were based on the energetic wellspring of the archetypal feminine.

Evidence of the first domestication of plants, which marks the Neolithic revolution, indicates that this began around 9000 B.C. Prior to this time, humans apparently lived in bands of gatherers and hunters in the time period known as the Paleolithic. While artifacts of the Neolithic clearly point to a worship of goddesses, those of the Paleolithic have such a striking similarity to the later work that archeologists now believe the religious orientation was the same. James Mellaart connects the art of the Upper Paleolithic of Europe with that of Neolithic Çatal Hüyük and Hacilar, which he discovered in the Anatolian plain.

> Çatal Hüyük and Hacilar have established a link between these two great schools of art and a continuity in religion can be demonstrated from Çatal Hüyük to Hacilar and so on till the great "Mother Goddesses" of archaic and classical times, the shadowy figures known as Cybele, Artemis, and Aphrodite. . . . The archeological, anthropological and artistic record of Çatal Hüyük is already strongly suggestive of an important heritage from the Upper Paleolithic . . . Upper Paleolithic art centered round the theme of complex and female symbolism (in the form of symbols and animals) shows strong similarities to the religious imagery of Çatal Hüyük. (Mellaart 1967, pp. 23, 24)

Archeologist Marija Gimbutas, in a seminar in San Francisco in 1987, noted that many identical images of the feminine occur from the Paleolithic into the Neolithic. With this evidence, we now have a 25,000-year continuous history of a religion oriented around the archetypal feminine. What is the impact of this long ancestral history on the psyche? The masculine-dominated religions of our era have a relatively short history of 3,000 or 4,000 years. The female religions which preceded them have left their imaginal imprints on the unconscious psyche, and these rich images surface in countless ways in dreams, fantasies, and creative work of present-day women and men.

What follows is an overview of the Neolithic cultures that preceded and then developed directly into Western civilization. I would like to ask you to listen to the descriptions of these societies as you would to a series of dreams.

James Mellaart made the first discoveries in 1957 in Turkey. Only one year before, the eminent archeologist, Seaton Lloyd, wrote:

> The region more correctly described as Anatolia shows no sign whatever of habitation during the Neolithic period. (Singh 1974, p. 65)

Mellaart first discovered the mound of Hacilar. A year later he found the spectacular city of Çatal Hüyük somewhat to the east. Çatal Hüyük is the largest Neolithic settlement discovered so far in

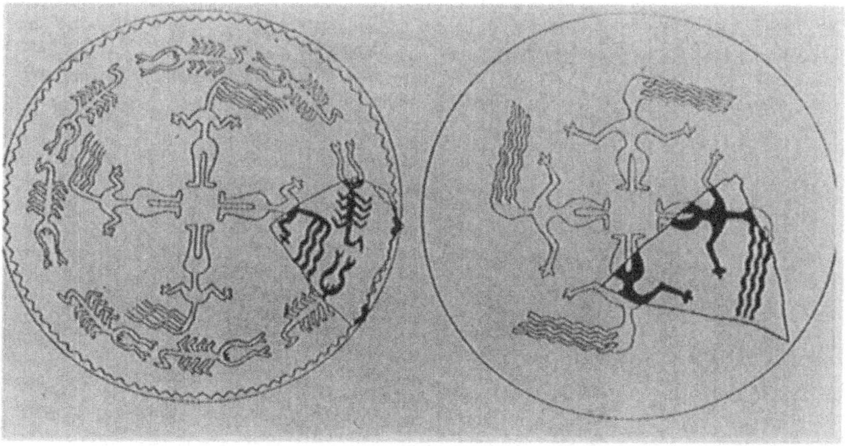

Figure 6. These goddesses with flowing hair and scorpions appeared on Samarran deep plates from northern Iraq (from Goff 1963, figures 32, 33).

the Near East. The culture was active between 6700 B.C. and 5700 B.C. Fourteen building levels have been uncovered, and virgin soil has not yet been reached. The people lived in a large town, perhaps 10,000 in population at its height. Houses were mud brick beehivelike structures with entrances through the roof. The large number of shrines in the housing structures is particularly noteworthy, one for every four or five homes in the portion now excavated.

The many shrines are elaborately decorated, giving us a vivid picture of the religion at Çatal Hüyük. The central figure in the worship is a goddess in many guises. She is the birth-giving goddess, legs spread wide, in her earliest image, a bas relief in plaster on a wall. Below her are rows of breasts formed over the beaks "of vultures, lower jaws of wild boar, heads of weasel and fox, all scavengers and harbingers of death" (Mellaart 1970). Beaks and jaws protrude from the red painted nipple. She is goddess of life and death, nourishment of the breast intimately united with the sharp bite of scarcity, misfortune, and death.

She appears as maiden alone, molded in clay on the shrine wall, dancing or running, her long hair streaming behind her. She appears in another wall sculpture as twin goddess, pregnant mother and pubescent maiden. In one fresco, a worshipper with face covered

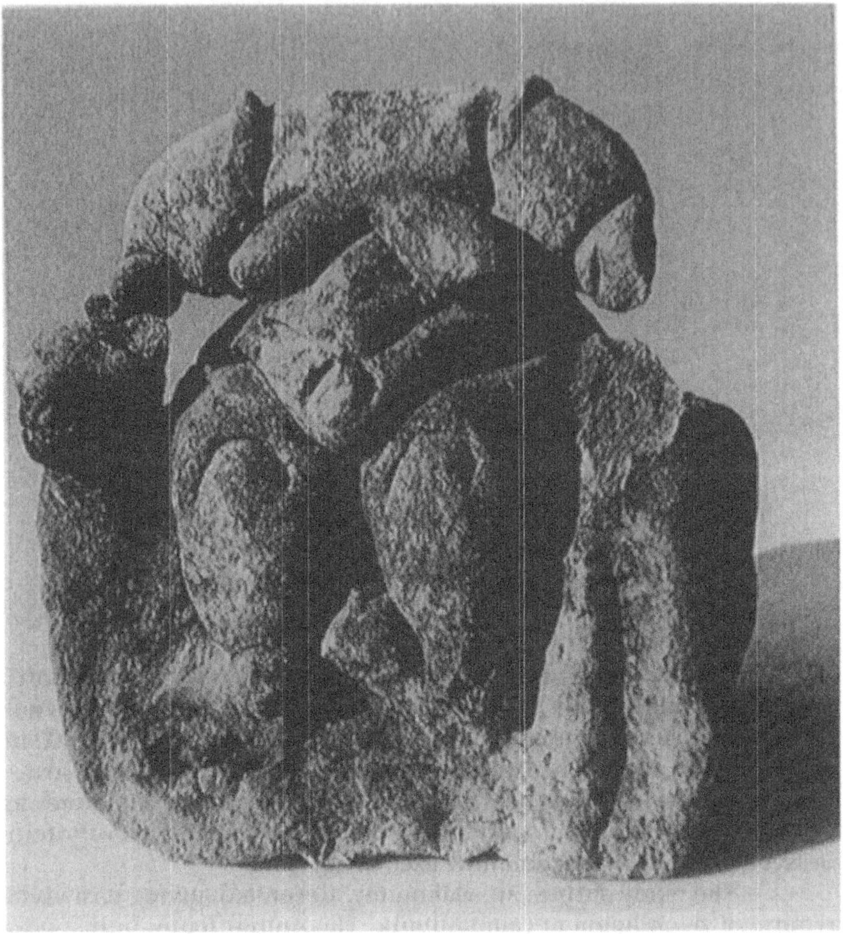

Figure 7. Goddess figurine giving birth on a throne with two felines as arm rests. From a grain bin of a shrine at Çatal Hüyük (from Mellaart 1967, p. 157).

approaches her as a triple goddess figure. Clay figurines of her appear in grain bins, as she is deity of crops. She is a huge figure molded on the wall of a shrine, watching over a scene painted on an adjoining wall of enormous vultures as they strip the flesh from the bodies of the dead. She encompasses all, life and death; all the vicissitudes of the natural world are held in her embrace.

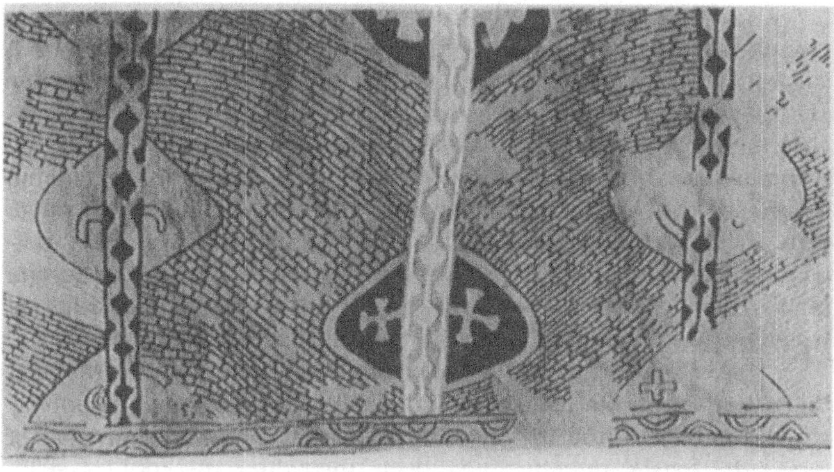

Figure 8. Kilim pattern painted in red, black, and white on a shrine wall, Çatal Hüyük (from Mellaart 1967, p. 89).

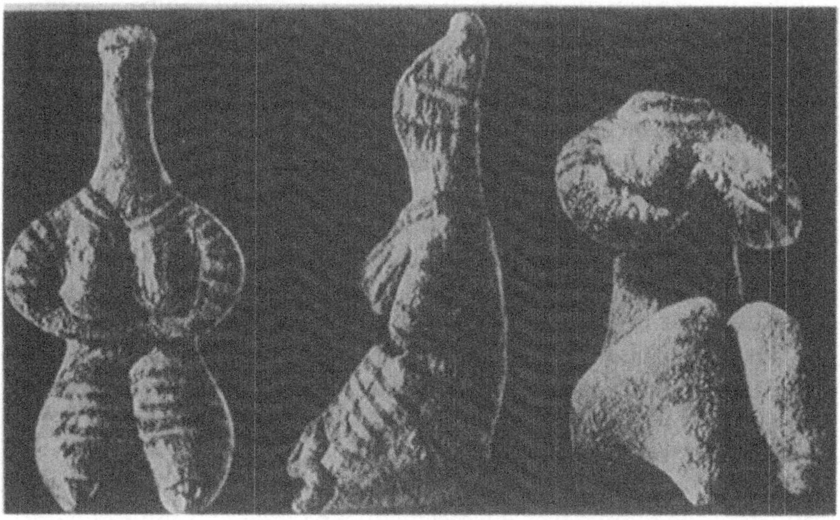

Figure 9. Mother goddesses painted with red stripes from Tell Halaf (a culture that was similar to Jarmo), northern Iraq (from Parrot 1961, p. 48).

This society evidently enjoyed a spirit of cooperation between women and men, and perhaps equality, although in excavated burial sites, it is apparent that women were given a more-honored status, and that priestesses outnumber priests. Mellaart believes women created the religion at Çatal Hüyük. Women's status was enhanced by their discovery of and control over agriculture. From the art-making tools found only in women's graves, excavators surmise that women were the artists, also. Çatal Hüyük gives us the earliest textiles, pottery, and basketry in the Near East. Elaborate designs of textiles are painted in the first frescoes on the walls of the shrines, paintings of weavings resembling the beautiful modern rugs from this area.

At Hacilar, Mellaart discovered a sizable Neolithic settlement that lasted about 800 years. Hacilar is noted for its exquisite pottery which developed from the style at Çatal Hüyük. A large number of terra-cotta female statuettes have been uncovered, the goddess seated, standing, enthroned, maiden, mature matron, pregnant mother, full-breasted nursing mother, mother with child, and mistress with animals. Many of these figures were found near the hearth in private houses (Mellaart 1970, p. 16).

South of Turkey, in present-day Iraq and Iran, lie many Neolithic village remains whose discovery and excavation began after World War II. According to archeologist Purushottam Singh (1974), numerous complex cultures existed side by side, distinguished by varying pottery and artifact styles and architectural remains. In Iraq, the extensive culture called after its principle site, Jarmo, yielded some 5,000 figurines, animal and human, including goddess figures with large buttocks and thighs. The Hassuna culture, with its distinctive pottery, developed skillfully modeled clay "mother-goddess" figures. At Choga Mami, excavated after 1966, archeologists found a new class of terra-cotta figurines. These goddesses are mostly standing with hands at the waist and have large exaggerated buttocks and feet. They are elaborately decorated with tattoolike markings on their faces, large slanted eyes, eyelashes and scalloped hair sculpted or painted on. Some have elongated birdlike heads. Choga Mami flourished around 4900 B.C.

Southern Iraq is the site of the important Neolithic culture of Eridu. Here the temple was successively expanded and built in eight levels, one over the other, from 5000 B.C. into historic time. Here we find the beautiful examples of the snake-headed goddess alone or nursing her snake-headed baby, her shoulders tattooed or marked with keloid scarring. From the Eridu culture came the Sumerians and the first examples of writing.

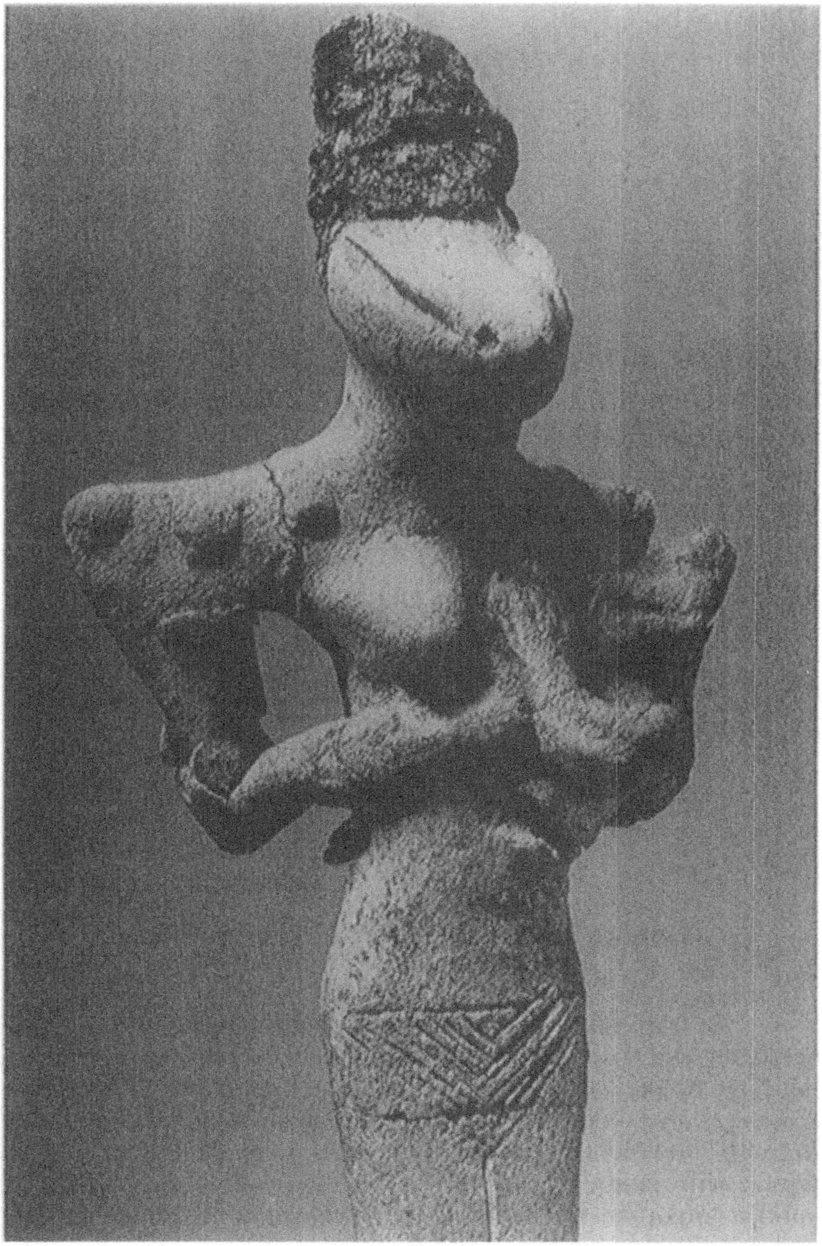

Figure 10. Snake-headed goddess nursing her baby, from Ur (from Parrot 1961, p. 59).

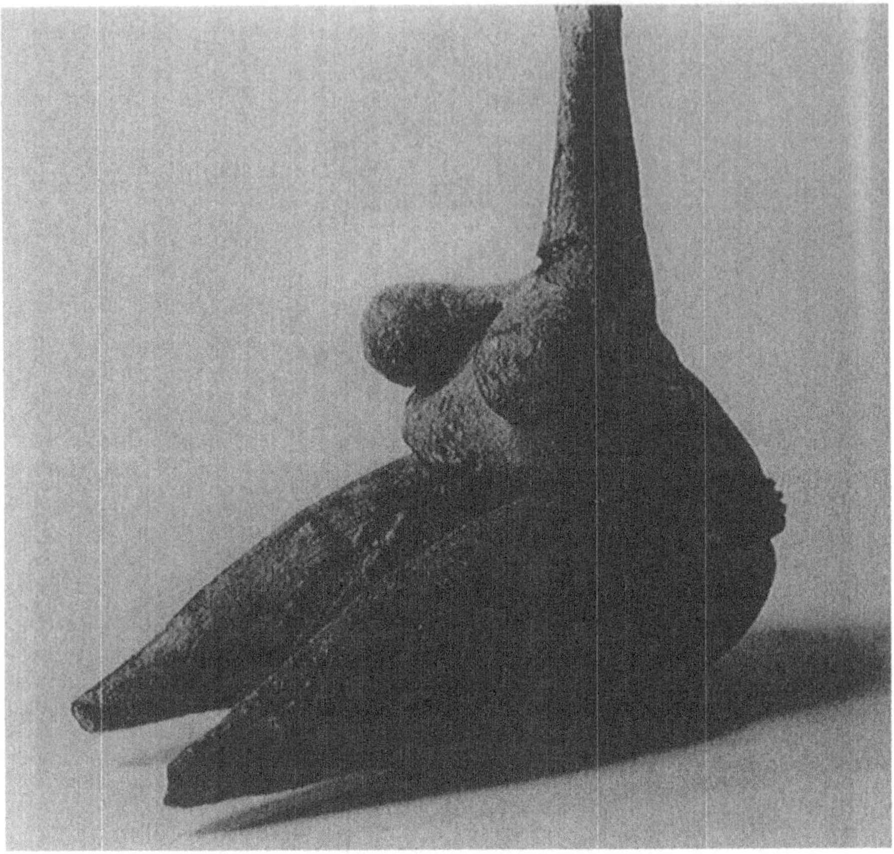

Figure 11. The Sarab Venus from Tepe Sarab, Iran.

In Iran, relics of prehistory came to light in 1949. At Tepe Sarab, diggers found the beautifully modeled Sarab Venus seated on her huge dolphin-shaped thighs, her large breasts protruding below an exaggerated long, slender neck. Ganj Dareh Tepe, a culture dating from 8400 to 6800 B.C., yielded figurines of a tiny, delicately modeled female with pointed head. At the 1963 excavation of Tepe Guran, another important site, workers found figurines of women and animals of stone, bone, and shell (Singh 1974).

In Iran, other sites of the Neolithic from 6000 B.C. to historical time yielded many mother goddess figures and other female fig-

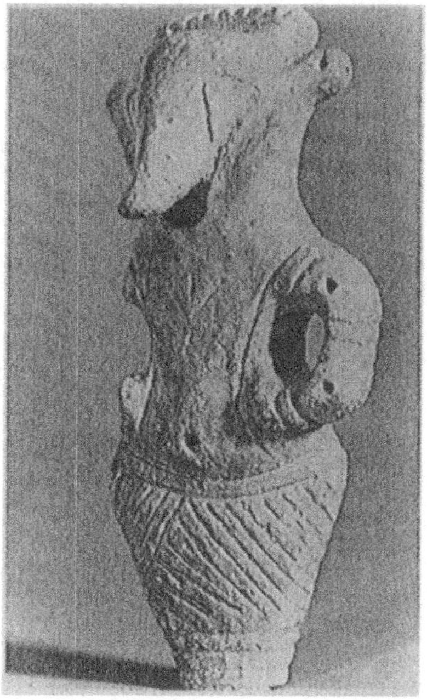

Figure 12. Bird goddess wearing a duck's mask and ritual skirt, Old Europe, fifth millennium B.C. (from Gimbutas 1982a, p. 139).

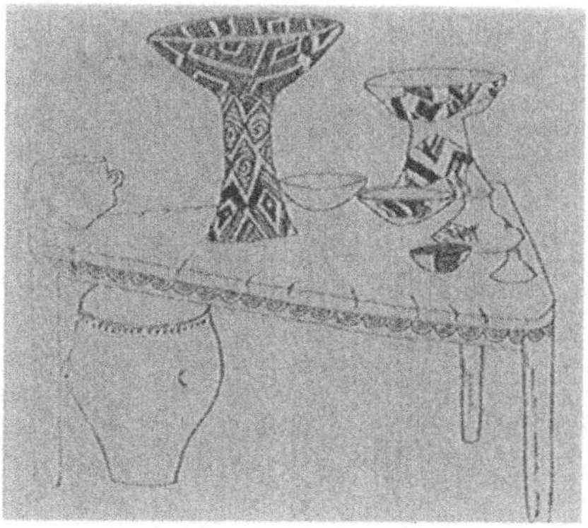

Figure 13. Drawing of a cult table with ritual pottery, Old Europe, fifth millennium B.C. (from Gimbutas 1982a, p. 81).

urines. At one particular site, Tepe Yahya, so far the only Neolithic site in southern Iran, in 1967, excavators uncovered, a very beautiful female figurine of green soapstone. She was lying on a bed of sixty-three flints together with three bone tools and three grooved whetstones, suggesting a shrine. Over this figurine there arose a debate that exemplifies the difficulty of overcoming a cultural bias in order to perceive objectively the reality of a very different culture. Was this a goddess figure, the excavators asked, or a phallus with breasts?

> It has been suggested that it represents the male phallus with the attributes of a female carved over it, but this view has been criticized by Carter who believes that the hole drilled in the top of the head was a purely functional device

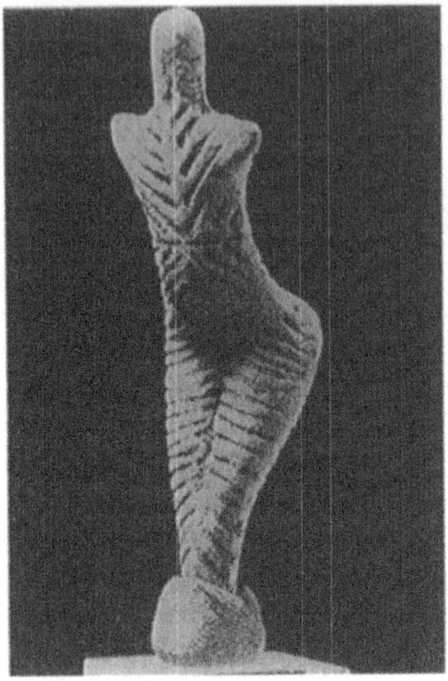

Figure 14. Bird or snake goddess with chevrons on front and back, Old Europe, fifth millennium B.C. (from Gimbutas 1982a, p. 141).

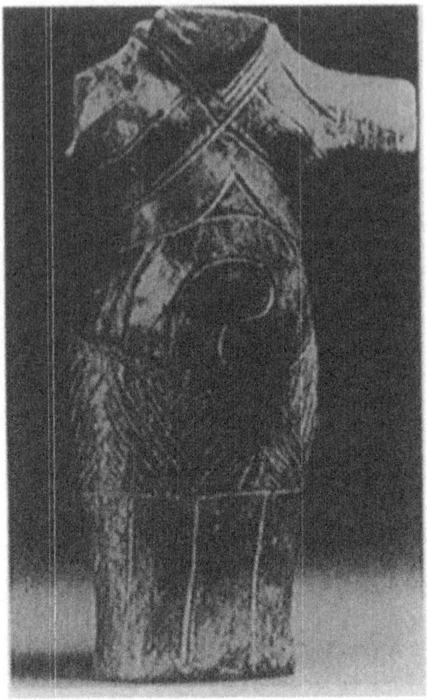

Figure 15. Pregnant goddess with a snake around her belly, Old Europe 5000-4500 B.C. (from Gimbutas 1982a, p. 202).

for fixing the attachment of hair or headdress and it is not the terminus of "the urethra" as suggested by the excavators. (Singh 1974, p. 195)

The third major area of Neolithic discoveries in the continuous line leading to Western civilization is Old Europe, about which archeologist Marija Gimbutas has written extensively (1982). This culture stretched from the Black Sea to the Adriatic, reaching its zenith around 5000 B.C. For several thousand years, the culture revolved around its religious core, the worship of goddesses. Some 30,000 sculptures have been excavated from 3,000 sites, representations of a goddess in two primary aspects. One is the goddess as giver of both life and death. In this aspect, she controls the length of the life cycle. At death, regeneration begins, so that death and regeneration are interwoven. The good and terrible mother is indivisible. The second aspect is the goddess as ruler of the fertility of nature itself. These two aspects of the goddess contain light and dark naturally and inevitably.

The cultures of Old Europe built elaborate temples to the goddess, some with roof openings through which she might fly, some in the form of her body. On the altars of the temples sat a rounded bread oven not unlike those in Pueblo villages of North America. Beside the oven stood a vertical loom. In a room below the sanctuary, the finest women artists created the sacred art of the culture which was dedicated to the goddess of the temple. As in Çatal Hüyük, the tools for making the exquisite vases and sculptures of Old Europe are found only in women's graves (Gimbutas 1982b, p. 9).

With the discovery of these early societies whose cultures moved energetically around the worship of goddesses, we begin to piece together a clear picture of a new pattern, a possibility for the individuation of women which we had formerly only intuited. The archetypal feminine begins to take a substantial shape and to have variety unknown before the discovery of these Neolithic cultures. A woman whose development takes her back to this feminine base as the orienting pattern for her ego sees life very differently from the woman grounded in the patriarchal culture's model for her sex. Truly this archetypal base is a goddess, not a phallus with breasts. Standing on this base, women no longer need to feel, "mother did not give me the desired genital, did not give me enough." The richness of these cultures as an expression of the archetypal feminine is a containing matrix for women, an archetypal ancestor to whom we may turn to inform our development and on whom we may ultimately fully rely.

This new consciousness presents the possibility of women's individuation process taking place outside Freud's paradigms. Connection to the feminine offers a wholly other source of energetic affirmation, a new/old archetypal pattern of identity. The reality of the goddess religions gives to woman a fully realized matrix in which her intuitive searching can now come to rest. No longer must she settle for an adaptation to the father, that identity which is forever secondary, forever unsatisfying. She now stands with the mother on female ground. Connection to the ancient female ancestors gives new meaning to May Sarton's search for precursors when, in a poem to Virginia Woolf, she said, "We go forward into the past" (Gilbert and Gubar 1988, p. 167). Truly women now can go forward under a new sign which flourished in the very ancient past.

What happened to obliterate this predominately peaceful tradition of goddess worshipers after so long a history throughout the Paleolithic and Neolithic? Gimbutas chronicles the repeated invasions and final destruction of Old Europe by the horse-riding, patriarchal pastoralists, the Kurgan (1983, p. 293). Remnants of the Old Europe culture appeared in the Aegean and survived on Crete and Cyprus for another 2,000 years. The rise of the patriarchy in Mesopotamia is credited to the destruction of clan kinship relationships as the organizing social principle (Rohrlich-Leavitt 1980, pp. 76-102), as well as to the military expansion of the state, the taking of captives, the invention of slavery, and the exchange of women (Lerner 1986). Later, in Judaism, the god Yahweh arose who was completely independent of nature, and while vestiges of the Canaanite fertility cult found a place within the Israelite religion, in the seventh century B.C., the last remains of the goddess religion were "mercilessly stamped out by Josiah, especially in his slaughter of the ritual prostitutes and the destruction of the Asheras" (Biale 1978, p. 10).

IV

Since we all grow up in a society with patriarchal values, we find the archetypal feminine primarily in the unconscious For a woman to return to the archetypal feminine as the matrix of her psyche, she must reorient through a connection to the unconscious feminine. This reorientation requires not only a resocialization into a female-based culture, but also requires a reinitiation through the major stages of female development. Such complete change may scarcely be possible in a lifetime. Nevertheless, many women in my practice have begun this process of reorientation led by strong supporting images from their dreams.

A forty-year-old housewife from a small country town, Barbara came into therapy seeking to adjust to the presence of her mother in her household. Barbara and her husband of twenty years had recently invited her mother to move in with them, since their two sons were now grown and gone. Barbara's smoldering hostility toward her mother was barely below the surface, conflicting with her caretaking self-image.

Barbara's initial dream was of a large house built around a beautiful tree. The tree's growth was beginning to crack the house structure and would soon destroy it altogether. The powerful image of the dream told me that Barbara's problem reached way beyond learning to cope with her mother. The tree as image of the Self and of her own individuation process was pushing her out of the psychological house of her adaptation to the culture, and that familiar house would necessarily come down. Indeed, this proved to be the case. Barbara soon asked her mother to move out. Not long after, with no warning, her husband abruptly left for another woman, an event I connected to the great disruption Barbara's emerging psyche caused the status quo.

Looking back from the perspective of Barbara's subsequent development, I can see that this initial dream revealed the tendency of her psyche's movement toward the archetypal feminine base. While the tree reaches toward the masculine spirit, it is grounded in the earth of the feminine. Sacred trees abound in the goddess religions. The tree is vegetative life and suggests movement in the psyche at a very deep, unconscious level.

Women who are making this move into a primary relationship to the feminine frequently bring an initial big dream pointing the direction. Sarah, a middle-aged housewife with three children still school-age, was in a twenty-year marriage when she came to me. Here is her initial dream.

> *On vacation with my husband and children, we suddenly realize an enormous volcano is erupting, spewing lava, but instead of fire, it spews golden sparks. They fill the air and threaten to fall on us. We seek shelter in a flimsy building. When I come out, my husband and youngest daughter have disappeared.*

From deep within the earth, the realm of the goddess, the golden substance of the Self shows forth, but as with the growing tree, the golden lava threatens to destroy the status quo. The movement of the psyche in both these dreams pictures a powerful, inevitable, natural force which takes the lead in the development of the dreamers, announcing a drastic change. A year into analysis, Sarah's husband also abruptly and unexpectedly left the marriage for another woman.

For myself as an analyst, this vision of women's psychological development casts a whole new light on women's dreams as they inform the process of development. With a woman client, I open myself as far as I can to the entire continuum of cultures, from the most fully developed woman-centered cultures to the most extreme male-centered cultures. Very soon the woman will tell me, through her dreams and her story, where she now sits on this continuum. When dreams of the feminine come, as they inevitably do, I see them not only as a needed compensation to a masculine-adapted woman, but also as a beckoning to this woman to begin the long journey back into the matrix of ancestral female orientation.

For all of us, our formative years in a patriarchal culture inevitably shaped an adaptation that is masculine. In addition to this masculine orientation, the women I see usually have one foot, at least, in paradise and have yet to face the reality of hardship, suffering, and death. Not that they haven't suffered, sometimes terribly, but they reveal a deep, perhaps unconscious hope or expectation that they will return to a primarily happy life after working out their troubles. Barbara was certain therapy could help her adjust to her mother's presence. This tenaciously held expectation of an idealized life usually covers a drastically wounded and rejected little girl.

In our work we as analysts travel with such women, providing a secure place for each of them to experience the pain and despair of the injury to the child they still carry. With this transition from a masculine base to a feminine in mind, I envision the injured child as not only being healed, but also discovering a vital, rich, nourishing, and sustaining matrix inside, which is the archetypal feminine. With this new feminine matrix, the analyst's hope that the woman may come to mother herself takes on new meaning. The mothering she may discover in herself is not only her image of good mothering within the patriarchal culture, but is the mothering of the matrifocal cultures whose ritual focus from birth to death is on the experience of being female. The archetypal feminine, as expressed in these cultures, holds her and honors her in her very particular female body and its potential for the powerful changes of menstruation, pregnancy, birth, breast feeding, child rearing, menopause, aging, and death, and all the metaphorical expressions of these states.

The analyst provides a place for the wounded child to be present and to be known. This child has lost contact with her female value as she adapted to a masculine-based culture. However, the child still carries female instinctuality, and beneath her wounds, she responds instinctually to the appearance of the feminine Self. This feminine Self appears in countless forms in women's dreams. With the recognition of a new feminine cultural base forming for women, I simply look at these images with a new slant. What does the Self want? Is this dream announcing an opening for the woman to travel out of her masculine orientation into this new world of the feminine?

Some dreams are very specific. The second year of Barbara's analysis, she dreamed of a group of women who do not believe in the moon.

I am outside at a religious ceremony. A woman leading carries a baby girl. A chorus chants to one side, a chant the baby taught the women. Two men, one black, one white, will teach this group, because the group does not believe in the moon. The men have a film to show, illustrating the reality of the moon. Inadvertently, the first of the film shows this group's church burning down. I am irritated that the men show this part of the film.

This dream is a call from the ancient female religions appearing in a modern dream as an available orienting matrix in the psyche of the dreamer. A new religious form is beginning, its liturgy being taught by a baby girl. New animus figures appear, black and white, carrying the opposites in apparent harmony and unity of purpose. The men will teach the group of women about the reality of the moon. These new animus figures relate to the archetypal feminine, not to the patriarchal masculine of her outer life adaptation. The dreamer, Barbara, shows her ambivalence to the change by being irritated that the men show in the film the old church burning down. Barbara, like many women, has lost her connection to cyclic time, moon time, and finds it hard to believe the psyche can be held in the waxing and waning, ebb and flow of the opposites. Moon time presents a new orientation based on her own lunar periodicity. She is called away from her old animus-dominated, factual orientation to an orientation based on the sway of the tides. She must learn this new view from supportive, knowledgeable, masculine figures.

The archetypal feminine Self is closely connected to moon time. Menstruation is the reminder in the woman's body of her belonging to the moon worshipers, of her deep grounding in cyclic time. For a woman out of touch with the feminine, dream images of the blood appear as dangerous aberrations of the normal flow. She dreams she is hemorrhaging or bleeding from her pores or passing large clots of blood. Such images can announce a readiness in the psyche to correct the imbalance and call the woman down into the feminine in her body.

One analysand dreamed repeatedly of aberrant menstrual flow. She had been raised in a strict Catholic family. During her first menses, she went to Mass and fainted. The conflict between the church of the fathers and the sacred blood of the mothers was too much for her sensitive psyche. After this incident, she made excuses to her parents to avoid Mass whenever she was menstruating. Her dreams of hemorrhaging dangerously called for a healing of her relationship to the feminine.

Women moving toward this new female base frequently dream early in analysis of a devastating calamity destroying the old way of living. Barbara dreamed a huge tree was growing through her house and threatened to destroy it. Sarah dreamed of a gold-spewing volcano. Earthquakes may shift the landscape. In one woman's dream, a fierce wind blows a strange tree spiraling into a harbor. Tornados bend and twist toward a dreamer's flimsy house where she cowers. The archetypal feminine announces herself through the elemental forces she controls—wind, storm, flood, hurricane, tornado, earthquake, fire. She destroys the old order, the old church, the old house, the old way of being with a sweep of her powerful hand. These forces of nature and their counterparts in the psyche—furies, rages, passions, intensities of emotion—announce the arrival of the goddess in her primal form.

Such primal natural forces are the familiar powers of the goddess and appear in women's dreams as a reminder of their ancestral heritage. The ancient poetry of Enheduanna, high priestess of Sumer in 2300 B.C., invokes this aspect of the goddess Inanna.

> Lady of elemental forces . . .
> flood-storm-hurricane adorned . . .
> a whirlwind warrior
> bound on a twister . . .
> a ditch of spilling water
> she floods over a road
> engulfs the one she loathes . . .
> fighting is her play
> she never tires of it
> she goes out running
> strapping on her sandals . . .

Judith Gleason, in her book on the goddess Oya, pleads for more understanding of women's passion.

> In being coached by compliant mothers to stifle rather than outride our storms, to dam and conceal our floods, to bank our fires and give tinder over to future husbands, the Oya in ourselves froze in its tracks . . . Thus, in other ways obstructed, Oya strikes us—quirking here, cramping there. Done with our brains, the indefatigable goddess goes jaggedly to work upon our bodies, cutting off circulation, opening sluices, instilling victims who could be votaries with a variety of "female complaints," catching them up in mindless swirls of activity, throwing them down into incapacitating vortices, playing havoc with appetite. Stop, Oya,

> we beg you! . . . We will strive to know your winds the better to reclaim our part of fire. (1987, pp. 18, 19)

While these elementary forces come early in analysis, they continue to infuse the more-developed woman with passion. Analysis calls the forces into livable containers. The raw forces are not lost. They ignite women's creativity. Gleason dares "to wrest women's fire back from Promethean culture-bearers":

> Unfortunately even Jung stereotypically categorizes the elements as active, creative, and masculine—fire and wind—as opposed to passive, submissive, and feminine—earth and water. Such identifications are culturally rather than archetypally determined and can lead to brainwashing in therapeutic situations that promise reclamation of the feminine. (1987, p. 30)

Feminine fire smolders unrecognized. "After a busy day the floor of the woman's therapy studio is strewn with drawings of incendiary vaginas and uterine cauldrons, burning with culturally imposed shame," says Gleason (1987, p. 31).

The analyst is challenged to open the door to these passions, to honor the dream images of storm and flood, earthquake and fire, as the raw materials of women's individuation. The wounded girl child has learned to conform and obey before she can experience the heat of her natural elements. Now the child within the woman is led through her dreams to a primal experience of the feminine in powerful, natural forms. First the woman must experience the intensity of her emotions before her stormy impulses can be transformed into channels of creativity.

This is the goddess. She is violent, randomly capricious, overwhelming, much larger than life. The process of analysis coaxes her energies into manageable expression, allows her fire to cook the wounded flesh of the psyche, transforming it into edible food. Or she allows herself to be impregnated, thus cooling the hot and bloody female force, allowing a softening to show forth. She is transformed, then, into gentle mother, birth-giving goddess, home center; but, as at Çatal Hüyük, the birth-giving goddess is never far from the breasts molded over the vulture's beak, or, as in Eridu, the gentle mother has the head of a snake and nurses her snake baby.

As women's individuation reconnects to the female past, women open to the interplay of elemental forces and their transforming containment, not in neat sequential doses but in unpredictable interaction, point and counterpoint, with which the woman wrestles the rest of her life. The woman who lives from the archetypal feminine base, then, travels expectantly from chaos to form and back to chaos again, just as her ancestors wove patterns out of a mess of threads which might easily at another time unravel. She is no longer the daughter protected from her passionate nature by the father's principles. Rather she is full woman, fully embracing the ebb and flow of her nature, as closely aware of the chaotic elemental forces as she is of their movement into creative containment.

Loosened by such cataclysms from the moorings of the patriarchy, the woman floats free but feels lost and bewildered. Sarah dreamed she was camping with a woman lover on the edge of a snowy wilderness filled with wild animals. Return to the natural world of the feminine can be harsh, cold, and terrifying.

At other times, the woman's dreams guide her and reassure her that her disorientation is a necessary part of discovering a meaningful new direction. In analysis, this is a time when she has big, archetypal dreams. She dreams she digs into the center of the earth or digs up old women's graves. There she finds weird animals or raging harpies. Or she finds strange reed posts on the fresh grave of a patriarchal analyst; the posts turn out to be the ancient symbol of the goddess Inanna. Or a swarm of bees fly spiraling upward out of an old record player. Or in a cave the ancient, decaying body of an old woman begins to move and rise. These archetypal images of the feminine are the ballast which give her stability in a time of confusion. It is important for the analyst to see the dreams as orienting signposts of the woman groping for connection to a feminine-based value system.

Adaptation to the culture imposes on most women a masculine-orienting frame which gives life meaning and predictability. The frame serves to guide her outer life in the absence of the development of consciousness of the feminine in her formative years. She becomes a phallus with breasts. The masculine frame is built over a lack, the absence of the feminine. She is terrified when this frame begins to fall away, for she senses the underlying void. When she becomes aware of the feminine structure that will catch her fall, she first recoils at its alienation from the culture. She dreams of the feminine as outcast, marginal, repulsive. She strongly resists giving up her favored and familiar status as daughter-captive to the fathers.

Recognition of the shadow is complicated by the fact that, in her allegiance to patriarchal values, this woman has repressed natural parts of her healthy instinctual growth, such as her full sexual womanhood and her assertive self-supporting voice. The analyst has to make a distinction in dream imagery between positive reemergence of the ancestral feminine and personal shadow issues. The feminine beckoning to this woman may appear shadowy since the woman still has the patriarchal perspective. One analysand dreamed of being seduced by a dark lesbian. Another woman dreamed a sexy blonde in a revealing red dress sat by her in church and made seductive advances. Both these images speak to the awakening in the dreamer's body of a traditionally forbidden sexuality. These images of the outcast or marginal woman reflect the dreamer's ambivalence toward the feminine rather than personal shadow.

These deep shadow issues arise between the values of the patriarchal god, Yahweh, who is wholly spirit and completely free of nature, and the values of the goddess, who is in and of nature and sanctifies the material world. The psychological conflict in woman centers on the body and its functions which are so intimately a part of her development. The patriarchal value of spirit over nature persists in one segment of the women's movement. This view stresses that women are "closer to nature" because of their burdensome bodies and are therefore less creative externally than men. Basing her argument on Simone de Beauvoir's influential book, *The Second Sex*, Sharon Ortner asserts that women's bodily functions are often the source of discomfort and pain. Breasts are irrelevant; menstruation uncomfortable, involving "bothersome tasks of cleansing and waste disposal." In pregnancy, "vitamin and mineral resources are channeled into nourishing the fetus, depleting her own strength and energies," and childbirth is dangerous and painful. Woman is doomed to mere reproduction of transient human beings, while the male creates lasting, eternal, transcendent objects (1974, p. 67).

The argument of de Beauvoir and Ortner that women are hampered in their ability to be creative by their bodily functions is the antithesis of the Neolithic goddess religions' belief that creativity issues from the female body. In the ancient religions, matter is the sacred and mysterious expression of the goddess. Women are created in her image, and the birth-giving and nourishing propensities of women's bodies match the goddess's fecundity and abundance. Not only are women's bodily functions not hampering of creativity, they are imbued with divine meaning; they inspired the exquisite art of the Neolithic and inform its ritual.

The frequent images of shame in women's dreams reflect this basic conflict between nature and spirit in the culture. The wounded child may long for the mother, but the masculine-adapted adult feels deep unconscious shame of her female body. This issue is present in dreams in which the female dreamer appears as a man. One analysand dreamed she was a black man in a jail. She is identified with the more-glorified masculine but remains an outcast in a prison.

The conventional shadow shifts in meaning as the woman experiments with new behavior. She may be outrageous, spilling over the boundaries of "appropriate" behavior. She must find her voice, as indicated in one woman's dream: she pulls a scream-stifling hand away from her mouth.

The goddess would have her tongue. Silence is tantamount to submission to the status quo. The goddess's insistence becomes more urgent. The woman remembers Inanna's use of her voice in Enheduanna's poetry:

> my Lady
> the blast of your voice
> crushes foreign lands . . .
> in splitting waves
> her shrill cries pierce
> Ebeh's failing heart. . . .
> her tongue's poison
> hurls a green-wilting curse
> over forest and fruit-bearing trees.

The tongue she seeks is not the cleverly adapted animus facility, but woman talk, a new language of women. Women's new language speaks in the creative inventions of Gertrude Stein, or in the work of the poet H. D., who says she writes from her "womb brain" (1982, p. 22). Contemporary theologian Mary Daly has put forth a new dictionary for women, *Wickedary* (1987), and Judy Grahn calls her lesbian and gay history *Another Mother Tongue* (1984). In Ursula Le Guin's story, "She Unnames Them," Eve takes away the names from all the animals, then gives back her own name, as she says to Adam:

> You and your father lent me this–gave it to me, actually. It's been really useful, but it doesn't exactly seem to fit very well lately. But thanks very much! It's really been very useful. (Le Guin 1986, p. 194)

While the woman utters the halting phrases of her newfound woman's language, her facile animus-adapted tongue is silenced. Her animus-inspired activities begin to feel like burdensome requirements. The basis of her way of being in the world is shifting.

Intrapsychically, there had existed an animus imprisonment.

Outwardly, the woman may have appeared highly adapted. It may have fooled even the analyst, because the woman looks entirely successful at work and love. Hidden, however, was the bewildered, injured child who still wonders why her budding female self was abandoned. No female ritual path led this child into the world of women, and somewhere deep inside she knows her true self is missing.

The feminine beckons to this little child, who still possesses the remnant of the female Self. It is this child who responds instinctively to the call of the archetypal feminine, for she longs for validation of her femaleness. She longs for the embrace of the mother, a new mother, not like her actual mother who also sleeps in the animus prison. When the injured child begins to respond to the healing approach of the Self, the woman begins to reconcile with her personal mother. One woman dreamed:

> *I am walking away from a glittering social event with my long-dead mother. I resolve to care for my old mother, take her home with me. I look down and see Mother's feet are broken and crippled, bound in the Chinese fashion.*

Only the appearance of the archetypal feminine Self can interrupt this repetitive inheritance of culture-bound adaptation. The analyst carries this healing Self in the transference. This enables the analysand to work with the injured child through her dreams and active imagination. The healing of the child becomes apparent as, in the analysand's image, the child grows older. Dream images appear set in the woman's childhood home, and healing interactions now take place where once there was violence, sexual abuse, and abandonment. One woman dreamed she found all of her beloved childhood dolls in a hidden closet. Another woman, after healing from a long series of dark depressions, dreamed the analyst appeared in her childhood home and taught her women's rituals.

The Self, which began the woman's long journey of return to female ground, now appears in dreams as priestess or female lover, guiding the woman through female initiation, awakening her deep love for women. The ritual initiations of matrifocal cultures become profoundly meaningful to her, as in this example: the Indians who lived in what is now San Diego County, California, dug pits for young girls when their menstrual periods first began. The women lined the pits with sweet-smelling sage, heated the pits with warm rocks. There in the pits the naked girls lay. The women placed a warm crescent-shaped stone between each of the girls' legs. For five days and nights, the old women sang the ritual songs and danced around the pit, imparting women's tribal wisdom to the young initiates.

Similarly, the woman in analysis dreams her own pubescent girl's initiation, no matter her actual age. The dreams of unnatural bleeding, which marked her alienation from the feminine, now subside, and dreams of bleeding herald a new awakening of love and respect for women's wisdom. One woman dreamed she was dancing with her granddaughter when suddenly she realized her period had started. The two of them went into the bathroom, and both cleaned the thick, red blood off her leg. The little girl bends to see where the blood comes from.

During this time of loving connection to the feminine Self, the woman notices a new masculine emerge in her psyche. Not only is the injured child healing and being led to womanhood, but a new animus is also growing out of the healed place. He may appear in dreams as a little boy, perhaps her own newly born boy baby. He may appear as an earthy man unlike the old image of hero, king, lawgiver, father. In one woman's dream, he was a cowherd. In Inanna's descent to the underworld, she is brought back to life by the life-giving waters and the life-giving plant of the earth god Enki. The sky gods refused to help her.

The new masculine supports her in her reaching out from the feminine, for he, like herself, worships the goddess, and in that respect, he is similar to men in matrifocal societies. He understands that she must "unname them," start fresh from a brand new perspective with new words for her experience. In Le Guin's story, Eve leaves Adam, says goodbye:

> "I'm going now. With the—" I hesitated, and finally said, "With them, you know," and went on out. In fact, I had only just then realized how hard it would have been to explain myself. I could not chatter away as I used to do, taking it all for granted. My words now must be as slow, as new, as single, as tentative as the steps I took going down the path away from the house, between the dark-branched, tall dancers motionless against the winter shining. (1986, p. 194)

No longer can the woman chatter away. She develops a new way of being in the world. Her awareness is deep and attentive, multilayered, and radiates in a circumference around her. She attends to the physical world through her body, takes the world in through all her senses. She no longer "names them" from her logos: tree, sky; rather she sees "dark-branched, tall dancers motionless against the winter shining." Just as when she is menstruating, she is attuned to her inner world while she goes forth in the outer.

I have watched many women go through this process of healing and self-discovery through reconnection to the archetypal feminine. I believe the energetic movement of the psyche in these women heralds a new opening in the cultural unconscious, which is bringing forth a new cultural form particularly relevant to women. Analysis is one of the few places in our culture that can guide a woman on this path, for women still have no truly female place nor time nor institution fully reflecting female nature. Because so many women are pushed from within to develop in this feminine direction, they will undoubtedly create spaces for their newfound orientation in the future. But at the present, a woman must search to find companions on the way.

How heartened we women are, then, to discover our ancestors. Reeling under the weight of past pain and present self-examination, we listen as Enheduanna tells us of other women who bore the struggle of individuation:[1]

those warrior women
like a single thread
come forth from beyond the river
do common work
in devotion to you
whose hands sear them with purifying fire

your many devoted
who will be burnt
like sun scorched fire bricks
pass before your eyes

And we join those before us who have sung her praises, understanding at last the poet's impassioned words:

your torch flames
heaven's four quarters
spreads splendorous light in the dark
you have realized
the queen of heaven and earth
to the utmost
you hold everything

---

[1]These two poems are from "Lady of Largest Heart."

entirely in your hands
your storm-shot torrentsdrench the bare earth
moisten to life
moisture bearing light
floods the dark
O my Lady
my queen
I unfold your splendor in all lands
I extol your glory
I will praise your course
your sweeping grandeur
forever

Queen
Mistress
you are sublime
you are venerable
Inanna
you are sublime
you are venerable
your great deeds
are boundless
may I praise
your eminence
O maiden Inanna
sweet is your praise

Bibliography

Biale, David. 1978. The god with breasts: el shaddai in the Bible. *History of Religions* 20:240–256.

Burkert, W. 1985. *Greek Religion.* Cambridge: Harvard University Press.

Colonna, M. 1980. Lilith, or the black moon. *Journal of Analytical Psychology* 25:325–350.

Daly, M. 1987. *Wickedary.* Boston: Beacon Press.

Freud, S. 1920. The psychogenesis of a case of homosexuality in a woman. *SE* 18.

________. 1931. Female sexuality. *SE* 21.

Gilbert, S., and Gubar, S. 1988. *No Man's Land.* New Haven, Conn.: Yale University Press.

Gimbutas, M. 1982a. *The Goddesses and Gods of Old Europe.* Berkeley, Calif.: University of California Press.

________. 1982b. Old Europe in the fifth millennium b.c. In *The Indo-Europeans in the Fourth and Third Millennia,* Edgar C. Polomé, ed. Ann Arbor, Mich.: Karoma Publishers.

________. 1983. An archeologist's view of PIE in 1975. *Journal of Indo-European Studies* 2:289–307.

Gleason, J. 1987. *Oya.* Boston: Shambhala.

Goetz, B. 1919. *A Kingdom Without Space* [*Das Reich ohne Raum*]. Potsdam: Constance, 1925.

Goff, B. L. 1963. *Symbols of Prehistoric Mesopotamia.* New Haven, Conn.: Yale University Press.

Grahn, J. 1984. *Another Mother Tongue.* Boston: Beacon Press.

_______. 1987. *Queen of Swords.* Boston: Beacon Press.

_______. 1988. Personal communication.

_______. In press. *Blood, Bread, and Roses.* Boston: Beacon Press.

Guntrip, H. 1968. *Schizoid Phenomena, Object Relations and the Self.* London: Hogarth Press.

Hall, N. 1988. *Those Women.* Dallas: Spring Publications.

Hamblin, D. J. 1987. Has the Garden of Eden been located at last? *Smithsonian Magazine* (May), pp. 127–129.

Harrison, J. E. 1962. *Prolegomena to the Study of Greek Religion.* London: Merlin Press.

H. D. 1982. *Notes on Thought and Vision.* San Francisco: City Lights Books.

Henderson, J. 1984. *Cultural Attitudes in Psychological Perspective.* Toronto: Inner City Books.

Irigaray, L. 1985a. *Speculum of the Other Woman.* Ithaca, N.Y.: Cornell University Press.

_______. 1985b. *This Sex Which Is Not One.* Ithaca, N.Y.: Cornell University Press.

Jung, C. G. 1919. Instinct and the unconscious. In *CW* 8:129–138. Princeton, N.J.: Princeton University Press, 1960.

_______. 1951. *Aion. CW*, vol. 9ii. Princeton, N.J.: Princeton University Press, 1959.

Kerényi, C. 1967. *Eleusis.* Princeton, N.J.: Princeton University Press.

_______. 1975. *Zeus and Hera.* Princeton, N.J.: Princeton University Press.

Koltuv, B. B. 1986. *The Book of Lilith.* York Beach, Maine: Nicolas-Hays.

Le Guin, Ursula K. 1986. She unnames them. In *Hear the Silence,* Irene Zahava, ed. New York: Crossing Press.

Lerner, G. 1986. *The Creation of Patriarchy*. New York: Oxford University Press.

Lessing, D. 1973. *Summer Before the Dark*. New York: Alfred Knopf.

_______. 1969. *The Four-Gated City*. New York: Alfred Knopf.

_______. 1975. *Memoirs of a Survivor*. New York: Alfred A. Knopf.

Mellaart, J. 1967. *Çatal Hüyük: A Neolithic Town in Anatolia*. New York: McGraw-Hill.

_______. 1970. The earliest settlements in western Asia. In *The Cambridge Ancient History*, I. E. S. Edwards, C. J. Gadd, and N. G. L. Hammond, eds. Cambridge: Cambridge University Press.

Mitchell, F. 1978. *Navajo Blessingway Singer*. Tucson: University of Arizona Press.

Ortner, S. 1974. Is female to male as nature is to culture? In *Women, Culture, and Society*, Michelle Rosaldo and Louise Lamphere, eds. Stanford, Calif.: Stanford University Press.

Parrot, A. 1961. *Sumer—The Dawn of Art*. New York: Golden Press.

Perera, S. 1981. *Descent to the Goddess*. Toronto: Inner City Books.

Rohrlich-Leavitt, R. 1980. State formation in Sumer and the subjugation of women. *Feminist Studies* 6:76–102.

Rose, J. 1986. *Sexuality in the Field of Vision*. London: Verso Press.

Stern, D. 1985. *The Interpersonal World of the Infant*. New York: Basic Books.

Singh, P. 1974. *Neolithic Cultures of Western Asia*. London: Seminar Press.

Wolkstein, D., and Kramer, S. N. 1983. *Inanna Queen of Heaven and Earth*. New York: Harper and Row Publishers.

Wyman, L. 1970. *Blessingway*. Tucson: University of Arizona Press.

Permissions

Figure 1. Photo by Gaye Williams. Reprinted by permission of the author.
Figure 2. Source: Samuel Weiser, Inc., York Beach, Maine 03910.
Figure 3. Source unknown.
Figures 4, 5, 7, 8. Permission requested from Thames and Hudson Intl. Ltd. and Professor James Mellaart, University of London, Institute of Archaeology.
Figure 6. Reprinted from B. L. Goff, *Symbols of Prehistoric Mesopotamia,* figs. 32 and 33. © 1963 Yale University Press, New Haven, Conn. Reprinted by permission of the publisher.
Figure 9. Source unknown.
Figure 10. Photo © Jean Mazenod, *L'art antique du Proche-Orient,* Éditions Citadelles & Mazenod. Reprinted by permission of the publisher.
Figure 11. Reprinted by permission of the author.
Figures 12, 14, 15. Source unknown.
Figure 13. Reprinted from Marija Gimbutas, *Goddesses and Gods of Old Europe: 6500-3500 B.C. Myths and Cult Images.* © 1981 Thames Hudson Ltd. Reprinted by permission of University of California Press.

Further information regarding unknown sources should be forwarded to Chiron Publications, 400 Linden Avenue, Wilmette, Illinois 60091.

Index

Made in the USA
Monee, IL
08 November 2026

67384907R00111